PROGRESS IN CLINICAL AND BIOLOGICAL RESEARCH

CONNECTIVE TISSUE RESEARCH
CHEMISTRY, BIOLOGY, AND PHYSIOLOGY

CONNECTIVE TISSUE RESEARCH
CHEMISTRY, BIOLOGY, AND PHYSIOLOGY

Proceedings of the VII European Connective
Tissue Clubs Meeting
Held in Prague, Czechoslovakia
September 8–11, 1980

Editors

Zdenek Deyl, PhD, DSc
Institute of Physiology
Czechoslovak Academy of Sciences
Prague, Czechoslovakia

and

Milan Adam, MD, DSc
Rheumatic Research Institute
Prague, Czechoslovakia

ALAN R. LISS, INC.   NEW YORK

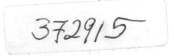

Address all Inquiries to the Publisher
Alan R. Liss, Inc., 150 Fifth Avenue, New York, NY 10011

Copyright © 1981 Alan R. Liss, Inc.

Printed in the United States of America.

Library of Congress Cataloging in Publication Data

Federation of European Connective Tissue Clubs.
    Connective tissue research.

    (Progress in clinical and biological research; v. 54)
    Bibliography: p.
    Includes index.
    1. Connective tissues — Congresses.
    I. Adam, Milan. II. Deyl, Zdeněk. III. Title. IV. Series. [DNLM: 1. Connective
tissue — Congresses.
    2. Collagen — Congresses. WI PR668E v. 54 / QS 532.5.C7 C752 1980]
QP88.23.F4   1981   599.01.852   81-954
ISBN 0-8451-0054-8   AACR2

Contents

Connective Tissue Research:
Chemistry, Biology, and Physiology, Page ix
© 1981 Alan R. Liss, Inc., 150 Fifth Avenue, New York, N.Y. 10011

Introduction

The editors feel that a brief explanation to the potential reader is in order. This volume is not intended to be an exhaustive treatment on connective tissue chemistry and biology. Neither is it simply a compilation of manuscripts resulting from a large international conference. We have tried to prepare a volume devoted to those branches of connective tissue research which are in the forefront of the scientific community at the present time. The papers were presented as plenary talks or introductions to workshops during the VIIth ECTC (Federation of European Connective Tissue Clubs) meeting in Prague (September 8–11th, 1980). The lectures were invited, and their selection was the result of discussions with the representatives of individual Connective Tissue Clubs throughout Europe. The editors and organizers of this meeting gratefully acknowledge this help. Special thanks go to Professor J. Scott of Manchester, England, and Professor L. Robert of Crèteil, France, for their interest, stimulating discussions, and highly qualified help.

Zdenek Deyl
Milan Adam

Prague, November 1980

Connective Tissue Research:
Chemistry, Biology, and Physiology, Pages 1-14
© 1981 Alan R. Liss, Inc., 150 Fifth Avenue, New York, N.Y. 10011

RECENT ADVANCES MADE IN INVESTIGATING THE MOLECULAR
STRUCTURE OF COLLAGENS

ROBERT W. GLANVILLE

MAX PLANCK INSTITUT für BIOCHEMIE

D-8033 MARTINSRIED,MÜNCHEN,WEST GERMANY.

Over the past 20 years,investigations on the structure
of the interstitial collagens,types I,II and III,
has led to a detailed knowledge of the primary
structure of collagen molecules (for review see
Glanville and Kühn 1979)and has contibuted to a
better understanding of collagen biosynthesis,
helix formation,fibre formation,crosslinking and
degradation processes.Amino acid sequences that
have been completed are the α1(I) chain from calf
and chick collagens and the α2 and α1(III)chains from
calf collagen.Both the human α1(III)chain and calf
α1(II) chain are near completion. The sequences of
the amino terminal extension peptides of calf
collagen proα1(I) and proα1(III) chains have been
determined, also the carboxy terminal extensions
of chick proα1(I) and proα2 chains, partly using
classical amino acid sequencing techniques and more
recently completed using neucleotide sequencing. The
amino terminal extension of proα2 and pre-procollagen
extensions are still under investigation.

Using the amino acid sequence of the triple
helical region of type I collagen,calculations have
been made to determine how molecules laterally and
axially aggregate to form fibres (Hofmann,Fietzek
and Kühn, 1978). The results are in good agreement
with those derived from Xray diffraction studies.
However, two models are still being discussed;one in
which five molecules form a microfibril and a second
in which the molecules are packed into a quasi hexagonal

structure. The formation of these higher structures
is a self assembly process which appears to have a
three step mechanism. The structure of the first
aggregate formed is still not clear and the role the
teleopeptides play in this process is unknown. The
structure of the lysine derived reducible crosslinks
in interstitial collagens have been elucidated (for
review see Light and Bailey 1979) but the nonreducible
crosslinks are still the subject of controversy.

Despite this detailed structural information,
there remain some important questions concerning interstitial collagens that have yet to be answered. It is
not known why an organism requires three interstitial
collagens. clearly typeII is cartilage specific and
the proportions of type I to type III in various
tissues is important, but why ? The primary and
higher strucures of these 4 collagen types are so
similar, it would be expected that one molecule
could substitute for another but this is not the case.
Secondly, the in vivo assembly of the collagen triple
helix is unclear. The mechanisms of chain selection,
association and helix formation still require
detailed investigation.

More recently, attention has turned to the
basement membrane collagens. These do not appear to
form fibrous structures, are very insoluble and ,
it was quickly realised, are pepsin sensitve. These
characteristics are atypical for collagens and it is
therefore expected that the collagenous structures in
basement membranes are formed following different
structural principles to those used for interstitial
collagens. In general, the function of the interstitial collagens is to bestow mechanical strength on
the extracellular matrix, this being done by forming
long fibres of various diameters, either in the form
of a meshwork (skin, bone) or parallel bundles
(tendon). However, basement membranes have different
functions depending upon the location of the membrane,
for example, as a filtration barrier (placenta,
kidney), scaffold in tissue repair and morphogenesis,
a receptor site for cell membranes (epithelial cells)
and as a support for the cytoskeleton of some cells
(fat cells). None of these functions requires that the
membrane has great mechanical strength. Whether the

collagenous components play an active role in the functioning of a basement membrane or only a passive supportive role is unknown.

The major structural components that have been isolated from basement membranes are type IV collagen, type V collagen, 7s collagen, laminin and fibronectin (for review see Timpl and Martin 1981). The latter two glycoproteins are non collagenous and will not be further described here.

7s collagen has a similar amino acid and carbo-hydrate composition to that of type IV collagen (low Ala, high Hyl, Leu, Ile, Phe. 22% carbohydrate mostly Glc-Gal-Hyl) but differs in that it contains 15 to 20 Cys residues and 10 to 15 Tyr residues per 1000 amino acids (Risteli et al 1980). The molecule, which contains two structurally distinct domains, has a molecular weight of 360 000 daltons. The bacterial collagenase resistant domain has a molecular weight of 225 000 daltons, a mid point melting temperature Tm of 70° and contains 42 to 45 Cys residues per 1ooo amino acids. The bacterial collagenase sensitive domain has a Tm of 42° and very little or no Cys. The molecule has a complex subunit structure as, when reduced, several fragments are produced with molecular weights in the range 30 000 to greater than 300 000 daltons as shown in figure 1.

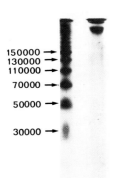

150000 →
130000 →
110000 →
70000 →
50000 →
30000 →

reduced (+)   (−) unreduced

Figure 1. Disc electrophorisis gels (5%) stained with coomassie blue, showing 7s collagen (long form) isolated from a pepsin digest of human placenta.

The origin of this molecule is still uncertain. It may represent a new type of collagenous structure or is perhaps the crosslinking region of a type IV collagen complex which has been fragmented by the action of pepsin during the solubilisation of basement membrane components.

Type V collagen is found in both basement membranes (Furthmayr et al, 1980) and in the extra-cellular matrix (Burgeson et al.,1976. Brown et al., 1978). It resembles more the interstitial collagens as it contains one third Gly, is a pepsin stable molecule with a length of about 3oo nm and has a Tm of 37°. It has the molecular formular $[\alpha 1(V)]_2\alpha 2(V)$ (earlier $[\alpha B]_2\alpha A$) but unlike interstitial collagens does not readily form fibrils. Many of the mammalian collagenases that cleave interstitial collagens do not cleave type V. As type V collagen has only been isolated from pepsin solubilised tissue, the molecule as it is found in vivo has not been characterised. It also remains to be seen whether there is a procollagen molecule with structural similarities to type I pro-collagen and whether crosslinking regions are present. A third chain that has been observed in some prepa-rations of type V, sometimes refered to as αC or $\alpha 3(V)$, has not been isolated as a native molecule and its relationship to type V is unclear (Sage and Bornstein 1979). The $\alpha 3$ chain appears to be tissue specific as demonstrated in figure 2.

Newly synthesised type IV collagen has been characterised in a number of cell and tissue culture systems (Tryggvason et al., 1980. Alitalo et al., 1980). After reduction and denaturation, two chains $\alpha 1(IV)$ and $\alpha 2(IV)$, have been identified with molecular weights of approximately 18o ooo and 165 000 daltons respectively. Although there does not seem to be any conversion of these products to smaller chains, it has not been possible to extract such products from basement membranes. The largest extractable chain described is 140 000 daltons and was isolated from a mouse tumor (Timpl et al.,1979). Because of the insolubility of basement membranes, it is necessary to solubilised their components using a proteolytic enzyme, usually pepsin. A typical preparation scheme

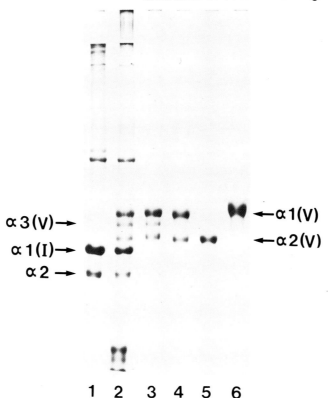

Figure 2. Stab electrophoresis gel (71/2%) stained with coomassie blue showing in lane 1, type I standard. Lane 2, pepsin solubilsed material from placental villi. Lane 3, type V isolated from material in lane 2. Lane 4, type V isolated from choreonic/ amneotic membrane of human placenta. Lane 5, α 2(V). Lane 6, α1(V).

for the collagenous components of human placental basement membrane is shown in figure 3. The type V, 7s and IV collagen fractions can be further purified by methods described in the literature (Bentz et al., 1978, Risteli et al., 1980, Glanville et al.,1979). The conditions for the first pepsin solubilisation are important as this determins the proportions of the various collagenous fractions and in the case of type IV collagen, the size of the fragments. To solubilise type V and 7s collagens, a temperature of

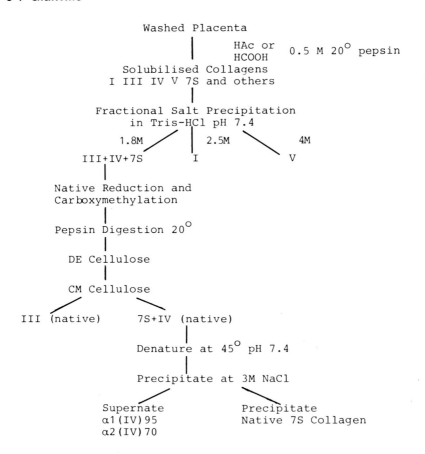

Figure 3. Scheme showing the separation of type V , 7s collagen and type IV collagen from pepsin solubilised human placental tissue.

20° and higher pepsin concentrations are necessary, whereas 4° pepsin solubilisation yields larger type IV collagen fragments but little type V and 7s. The size of the type IV fragments produced vary also with the animal species and tissue used. Such variations are illustrated in figure 4 for human placenta and bovine lens capsule type IV collagen prepared at 4° and 20°.

HUMAN PLACENTA

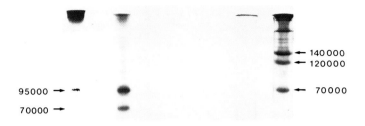

95000 →
70000 →

140 000
120 000

70 000

(−)   (+)   (−)   (+)
   20°   4°

BOVINE LENS CAPSULE

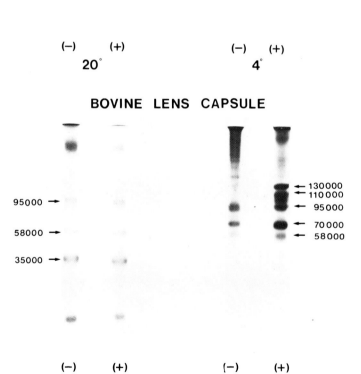

95000 →

58000 →

35000 →

130 000
110 000
95 000

70 000
58 000

(−)   (+)   (−)   (+)
   20°   4°

Figure 4. Disc electrophoresis gels (5 %) stained with coomassie blue showing pepsin fragments of type IV collagen isolated from human placenta and bovine lens capsule. The 20° pepsin solubilisation was carried out as shown in figure 3. In the 4° solubilisation, the native reduction, carboxymethylation and second pepsin digestion were omitted. (+) reduced (−) unreduced

Table 1 lists the pepsin fragments of type IV collagen that have been described in the literature and indicates the chain of origin of these fragments. It can be seen that fragments of approximately 140 000, 95 000 and 50 000 daltons form the α1(IV) chain have been isolated from many tissues and similarly 12o 000, 95 000, 75 000 and 5o ooo fragments from α2(IV) chain. This indicates that the type IV collagen in these tissues are structurally related. Mouse tumor and chick fragments are an exception to this generalisation as the major products appear to be around 50 000 daltons with no 95 000 or 70 000 dalton fragments.

Using the structural information available from investigations on human placenta, mouse tumor and bovine lens capsule type IV collagens, the pepsin fragments can be approximately aligned as shown in figure 5 .

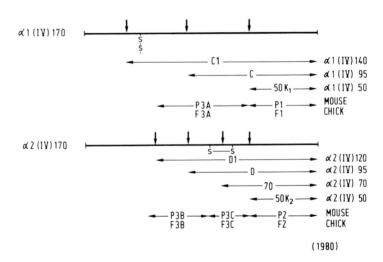

(1980)

Figure 5. Scheme showing the alignment of human and bovine type IV collagen pepsin fragments in relation to the intact α(IV) chains. Nomenclature used in the literature is shown between the arrows and the fragment size to the right. Mouse and chick fragments are included for comparison. ⬇ indicates the major pepsin cleavage sites.

Tissue	α 1 (IV)			α 2 (IV)				Authors
Human placenta	170K	100K				70K		Bailey, A.J., Simms T.J., Duance, V.C. and Light,N.D.
	140K	100K	70K-I			70K-II		Sage,H., Woodbury,R.G. and Bornstein, P.
		α(IV)95K α"(IV)95K				α'(IV)70K		Glanville,R.W., Rauter,A. and Fietzek,P.P.
	C'(140)	C(95)	50K₁		D(95K)	80K	50K₂	Kresina,T.F. and Miller J.M.
Lens capsule		α1(IV)95K						Dehm,P. and Kefalides,N.A.
	C-1(140K)	C(95K)	50K₁		D(95K)	80K	50K₂	Gay,S. and Miller,E.J.
	130K	C(95K)				D(75K)		Dixit,S.N. and Kang,A.H.
					85K	68K		Schwartz,D., Chin Quee,T. and Veis, A.
Kidney	140K	100K		D-1(120K)	D(95K)	80K		Tryggvason,K. and Kivirikko,K.I.
	C-1(140K)	C(95K)		D(140K)	B(93K)	75K		Dixit,S.N.
	C(140K)	A(93K)						Daniels,J.R. and Chu,G.H.
Mouse tumor	140K	P1(60K)					P2(50K)	Timpl,R., Bruckner,P. and Fietzek, P.P.
Chick		F1(53K)					F2(50K)	Mayne,R. and Zettergren,J.G.

Table 1. Pepsin derived basement membrane collagen fragments from various sources as reported in the literature. The fragments are grouped according to the chain of origin, α 1 (IV) or α 2 (IV). The numbers are molecular weights in kilodaltons.

Amino acid sequence analysis of pepsin and cyanogen
bromide fragments of mouse tumor and human placenta
type IV collagens have revealed the presence of non
triple helical interuptions as shown in figure 6.
The lengths of the non helical sequences are vaiable
and the frequency of occurance of these regions along
the α chains is still unknown. It was also surprising
to find almost identical sequences, which also contained non helical regions, in peptides from mouse
and human origin (Figure 6: P2 and E, CB 5 and CB 6).
This indicates that, despite the differences in
pepsin fragmentation patterns observed, there are at
least some regions of mouse tumor type IV which are
homologous to human type IV. It is too early to discuss
the significance of the non helical interuptions but
clearly these will have a profound effect upon the
structure and function of the collagen molecule in
basement membranes.

Although our knowledge of the collagenous
components of basement membranes has increased
tremendously in the last 4 years, there remain a
number of basic questions still unanswered. How many
type IV collagen molecules are there $[\alpha 1(IV)]_3$,
$[\alpha 2(IV)]_3$ or $[\alpha 1(IV)]_2 \alpha 2(IV)$ and how large are
these chains in vivo? Is there a type IV procollagen?
What is the relationship between 7s collagen and
type IV ? Are there other, as yet poorly characterised
collagen molecules in basement membranes ('C' chain
of type V, α3 from mouse tumor, epithelial
collagen). In an attempt to answer some of these
questions, extensive primary structural investigations
of the collagenous components of basement membranes
will be necessary.

Pepsin fragments

Human α1(IV)95   Tyr-Phe-Asp-Leu-Gly-Leu-Gly-Gly-Asp- Y -Gly-
       α2(IV)70   Glu-Ala-Ile-Gln-Pro-Gly-Glu-Ile- Z -Gly-Pro- Y -Gly-Leu-Hyp-Gly-
       D   Glu-Ala-Ile- Z -Gly-Leu-Hyp-Gly-Leu-Hyp-Gly-Pro-Hyp-Gly-Phe-Ala-
       E   Pro-Gly-Met- Z -Asp-Ile- Z -Gly-Glu-
       F   Tyr-Gly-Ile-Gly-Ala-Thr-Gly-Asp-Phe-Gly-Asp-Ile-Gly-Asp-Thr-
                   Ile-Asn-Leu-Pro-Gly-Arg-Hyp-Gly-Leu- Y -Gly-Glu-Arg-Gly-Thr-Thr-
                   Gly-Ile-Hyp-Gly-Leu- Y -Gly-

Mouse P1   His-Val-Asp-Met-Gly-Ser-Met-Gly-Gly-Gln-Gly-Gly-Asp-Gln-
       P2   Pro-Gly-Met-Lys-Asp-Ile- Z -Gly-Glu- Y -Gly-Asp-Glu-Gly-

Cyanogen bromide peptides

Human CB6   Gly-Pro-Hyp-Gly-Pro-Gln-Gly-Gln-Pro-Gly-Gly-Hyp-Gly-Ser-Hyp-Gly-
                   Z -Ala-Thr-Glu-Gly-Pro-

Mouse CB5   Gly-Pro-Hyp-Gly-Pro-Gln-Gly-Gln-Hyp-Gly-Gln-Hyp-Gly-Leu-Hyp-Gly-Thr-Hyp-Gly-
                   Z -Pro-Val-Glu-Gly-Pro-

Figure 6. Amino acid sequences of pepsin fragments and cyanogen bromide peptides
from human placenta and mouse tumor basement membrane (type IV) collagens. Non
helical regions are underlined. Y represents probable glycosylated hydroxylysine
residues. Z represents unidentified residues in non helical regions which may
also be glycosylated hydroxylysine. Mouse P1 and P2 sequences are taken from
Timpl, Bruckner and Fietzek, 1979 and mouse CB5 from Schuppan, Timpl and
Glanville, 1980.

References

Alitilo K, Vaheri A, Krieg T and Timpl R (1980).
Biosynthesis of two subunits of type IV procollagen
and of other basement membrane proteins by a human
tumor cell line. Eur J Biochem 109:247.

Bailey A J, Sims T J, Duance V C and Light N D (1979).
Partial characterization of a second basement
membrane collagen in human placenta. FEBS Lett 99:361.

Bentz H, Bächinger H P, Glanville R W and Kühn K (1978).
Physical evidence for the assembly of A and B chains
of human placental collagen in a single triple helix.
Eur J Biochem 92:563.

Brown R A, Shuttleworth C A and Weiss J B (1978).
Three new α chains of collagen from a non basement
membrane source. Biochem Biophys Res Commun 80:866.

Burgeson R T, El Adli F A, Kailila I and Hollister D W
(1976). Fetal membrane collagens: identification of
two new collagen alpha chains. Proc Nat Acad Sci USA
73:2579.

Daniels J R and Chu G H (1975). Basement membrane collag
of renal glomerulus. J Biol Chem 250:3531.

Dehm P and Kefalides N   (1978). The collagenous
component of lens basemant mambrane; the isolation
and characterisation of an α chain size collagenous
peptide and its relation to newly synthesised lens
components. J Biol Chem 253:6680.

Dixit S N (1979). Isolation and characterisation of
two polypeptide chains C and D from glomerular basement membrane. FEBS Lett 106:379.

Dixit S N and Kang A H (1980) Basement membrane collager
cyanogen bromide peptides of the D chain from porcine
kidney. Biochemistry (1980) 19:2692.

Gay S and Miller E J (1979). Characterisation of lens
capsule collagen: evidence for the presence of two
unique chains in molecules derived from major basement membrane structures. Arch Biochem Biophys 198:37(

Glanville R W, Rauter A and Fietzek P P (1979).
Isolation and characterisation of a native placental
basement membrane collagen and its component α chains
Eur J Biochem 95:383.

Glanville R W and Kühn K (1979). The primary structure
of collagen.In Parry DAD, and Creamer LK (eds):
"Fibrous Proteins: Scientific, Industrial and Medical
Aspects," Academic Press, London and New York, P 133.

Hoffmann H, Fietzek P P and Kühn K (1978). The role
of polar and hydrophobic interactions for the molecul

packing of type I collagen: A three-dimensional evaluation of the amino acid sequence. J Mol Biol 125:137.

Kresina T F and Miller E J (1979). Isolation and characterisation of basement membrane collagen from human placental tissue. Evidence for the presence of two genetically distinct chains. Biochemistry 18:3089.

Light N D and Bailey A J (1979). Covalent crosslinks in collagen. In Parry DAD, and Creamer LK (eds):"Fibrous Proteins: Scientific, Industrial and Medical Aspects," Academic Press, London and New York,P 151.

Mayne R, Zettergreen J G (1981). Type IV collagen from chick muscular tissues. Isolation and characterisation of the pepsin resistant fragments. Biochemistry 19:4065

Risteli J, Bächinger H P, Engel J, Furthmayr H and Timpl R (1980). 7S collagen : characterisation of an unusal basement membrane structure. Eur J Biochem 108:239.

Roll J F, Madri J A, Albert J and Furthmayr H (1980). Codistribution of collagen type IV and AB_2 in basement membranes and mesangium of the kidney. J Cell Biol 85:597.

Sage H and Bornstein P (1979). Characterisation of a novel collagen chain in human placenta and its relationship to AB collagen. Biochemistry 17:3815.

Sage H, Woodbury R G and Bornstein P (1979).Structural studies on human type IV collagen. J Biol Chem 254:9893.

Schuppan D, Timpl R and Glanville R W (1980). Discontinuities in the triple helical sequence Gly-X-Y of basement membrane (type IV) collagen. FEBS Lett 115:297.

Schwartz D, Chin-Quee T and Veis A (1980).Characterisation of bovine anterior lens capsule basement membrane collagen. Eur J Biochem 103:27.

Timpl R and Martin G R (1981). Structural components of basement membranes. In Furthmayr H (ed)"Immunochemistry of the extrcellular matrix. Vol I Methods CRC Press Inc. in press.

Timpl R, Martin G R, Bruckner P, Wick G and Wiedemann H (1978). Nature of the collagenous protein in a tumor basement membrane. Eur J Biochem 84:43.

Timpl R, Bruckner P and Fietzek P P (1979). Characterisationof pepsin fragments of basement membrane collagen obtained from a mouse tumor.Eur J Biochem 95:255.

Tryggvason K and Kivirikko K I (1978).Heterogeneity
   of pepsinsolubilised human glomerular basement membran
   collagen . Nephron 21:230.
Tryggvason K, Robey P G and Martin G R (1980).
   Biosynthesis of type IV procollagens. Biochemistry
   19:1284.

Connective Tissue Research:
Chemistry, Biology, and Physiology, Pages 15-44
© **1981 Alan R. Liss, Inc., 150 Fifth Avenue, New York, N.Y. 10011**

CHROMATOGRAPHIC AND ELECTROPHORETIC METHODS FOR COLLAGEN
SEPARATION

Z. Deyl, M. Horáková and M. Adam

Inst of Physiology Czech. Acad. Sci. and
Res. Inst. Rheum. Diseases,
Prague, Czechoslovakia.

It is really worth while to overlook after years the
time that has elapsed since the first attempt to survey
human's knowledge on a particular topic was done. With collagens and connective tissue proteins even books on methodology are available today (Hall, 1976) that make us hardly
believe the tremendous progress that we are witnessing in
collagen separations. When, some fifteen years ago, together
with the late Jan Rosmus we were preparing the first review
on chromatographic and electrophoretic methods of collagen
separation, the techniques were restricted to Sephadex chromatography (a rather unsuccessful separation), to (today
classical) carboxymethylcellulose separation of Piez et al.
(1963), and the fashion of the day was to separate collagen
polypeptide chains by polyacrylamide gel electrophoresis.
In the subsequent years separation procedures, i.e. chromatography and electrophoresis,developed considerably and their
progress was adequately reflected in the separation procedures
used in collagen chemistry. It is, perhaps, justified to say
that the progress in separation methods contributed to the
discovery of collagen polymorphism and to the more detailed
description of individual collagen and procollagen species.
We attempted, therefore, to summarize the methods available
today for the separation of collagen proteins with the hope
that such a survey will help the newcomers to orient themselves in the field and the experienced ones may get some
additional inspiration from such a review.

Generally saying mainly two types of liquid column
techniques are used for collagen separations: gel permeation
chromatography which is exploited for the separation of indi-

vidual chain polymers and ion exchange chromatography that is applied for the separation of individual chain species. It is, perhaps, not surprising that the first category of separations is done with denatured molecules while native molecules are separated by ion exchange chromatography. In the latter case, however, separations of denatured poly- peptide chains are used as well in specialized situations. The separation efficiency of conventional methods that are most popular is not sufficient and therefore several chro- matographic steps (resembling multidimensional chromato- graphy, based on combination of the above mentioned principles) are necessary to obtain purified materials. The domain of current separations are preparative procedures; much less has been done on the analytical scale, but with the new, high efficiency separations the proportions are likely to change.

Detection of collagens during chromatography is done by absorbancy measurement at 230 nm (because aromatic residues are nearly absent in the structure) or, if fractions are taken, by hydroxyproline assay. In the latter case aliquiots of each fraction are taken for quantitating the collagen specific amino acid. Recently a variation of the classical method of Stegemann (1958) was published (Huszar et al. 1980): samples of collagen are hydrolysed in alkali, acidified and the hydrolysate is let to react with p-dimethylamino benzaldehyde in the presence of perchloric acid and chlor- amine T. After fifteen min reaction time the color yields are read at 550 nm.

Both direct measurement at 230 nm and hyp detection have their advantages and drawbacks. The direct O.D. re- cording is sensitive, but selectivity is low as all peptides absorb at this wavelength. Also, solvents or reactants absorbing at this wavelength cannot be used (β-mercapto- ethanol). On the other hand the specificity of the hyp assay is much higher. The method itself has not been however, adapted to work on-line and thus it can be used with the perspective high-efficiency techniques only with some dif- ficulties.

As far as electrophoretic separations is concerned so far the best results were obtained with slab gel electro- phoresis. It is recommended to use gradient gels. Staining and destaining of gels is conventional. It should be emphasized that in collagen separations electrophoresis in

acid pH without SDS and in alkaline media in the presence
of the detergent offer nearly the same results. Because
of the close relation between individual collagen species
and because of the neglegible charge differences between
individual collagen α-chain polymers, focusing methods are
without perspectives.

CHROMATOGRAPHIC SEPARATIONS

Separation of collagen type I and III

Since type III collagen is present exclusively in the
insoluble collagen fraction, limited proteolysis of insoluble collagen is an inevitable step in analysis. This yields,
however, a mixture of collagen type I (originally heavily
cross-linked), type III and a considerable amount of contaminating proteoglycans.

Separation of collagen type I and III can be done either
with purified material from which contaminats were removed
(Adam et al., 1979) or with crude mixtures arising after
partial proteolysis.

In the first procedure proteoglycans are removed by
DEAE-cellulose chromatography. It should be stressed that
removal of proteoglycans is essential for subsequent isolation of collagen type III by both the Bio-Gel A-1.5 m chromatography and the salting-out method. The first fraction
containing purified collagen is dialyzed and used for further separation, the other (proteoglycan) fraction is
discarded.

The next step is the second DEAE-cellulose chromatography in which a combined peak of collagen types I and III
is separated from the bulk of other collagen types (Fig. 1).
It is advisable to attempt the separation of collagen type
I and III from other collagen types and proteoglycans in a
separate chromatographic run as otherwise clear separations
of individual collagen types are obtained only with dif-
ficulties. The first peak in this separation is formed by
collagen types I and III; the peak eluted after the gradient
has been introduced is mainly collagen type V.

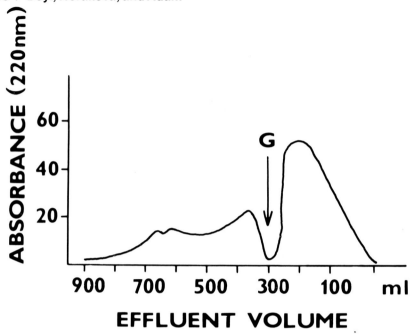

Fig. 1. DEAE-cellulose chromatography of a collagen mixture.
Eluting buffer: 0.02 M NaCl-0.05 M Tris-HCl, pH 7.5, 2 M
with respect to urea. G indicates the beginning of the
linear gradient (0.02-0.3 M NaCl in 0.05 M Tris-HCl, 2 M with
respect to urea, twice 500 ml); 2.5 x 20 cm column.

The separation of collagen types I and III is based on
the difference in rel. mol. mass after pepsin digestion.
Thus separation can be a chieved by two subsequent chromato-
graphies on Bio-Gel A-1.5 m. The second run is used to get
products of high purity. In the first run the UV-absorbance
profile exhibits three maxima corresponding to 300 000,
200 000 and 100 000 relative molecular mass. Contrary to the
previous separation procedure (DEAE-cellulose chromatography)
this one is carried out with denatured collagen. Samples
are heated to 43° to ensure denaturation before application
to the column. Due to the disulphide bonds, collagen type
III is present in the fastest peak, where chain polymers of
collagen type I are present as contaminants. Peak with
higher retention volume contains depolymerized collagen type
I (Fig. 2).

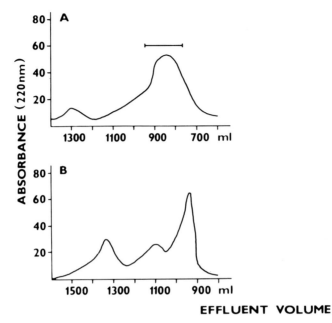

Fig. 2. Bio-Gel A-1.5 m chromatography. (A) A mixture of
collagen types I and III (isolate from the second DEAE-
cellulose chromatography). Eluting buffer: 1 M CaCl$_2$ in
0.05 M Tris-HCl (pH 7.5) and 2 M urea. The dominant peak
represents chain polymers of collagen type I + III; the
small peak contains single collagen chains (type I). (B)
Rechromatography of the dominant peak from the run in (A) as
indicated by the horizontal bar, after reduction and alkylation. Eluting buffer identical with that of (A). Peaks from
right to left: γ-fraction (chain polymers, a mixture of
types I and III cross-linked with non-reducible cross-links),
single polypeptide α chains.

    Equally good separations are obtained with Bio-Gel A-5 m.
No preliminary purification is necessary, as alternatively
to the above procedure most of the contaminating substances
can be removed during the chromatographic procedure itself
by using a buffer that is 2 M with respect to guanidine
(Klein and Chandrarajan, 1977).

    The final separation of type I and III can be done also
by making use of Sepharose CL6B. In the method suggested
by Chandrarajan and Klein (1980) the separation can be done

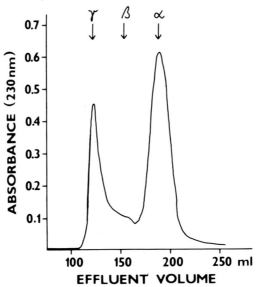

Fig. 3. Separation of type I(α) and type III(γ) collagens by molecular sieve chromatography on a Sepharose CL-6B column (210 x 1.6 cm). The sample was eluted with 2 M guanidine HCl-0.05 M Tris-HCl (pH 7.5) at room temperature. Detection by O.D. monitoring at 230 nm.

directly by molecular sieving of the pepsin treated material without previous purification. This is because most of the contaminating material (proteoglycans) is removed by heat denaturation in 2 M guanidine hydrochloride prior to separation which serves also to remove last traces of pepsin that might coprecipitate with the limited proteolysis solubilized material. Other denaturing agents like urea or $CaCl_2$ are supposed to be unsuitable because along with the solubilization of collagen proteins they also solubilize deantured pepsin (Chandrarajan and Klein, 1980) (Fig. 3).

The use of a longer column (210 cm) of the cross-linked agarose appears necessary to obtain separations comparable to those achieved on shorter (115 cm) column of non-cross-linked agarose (Klein and Chandrarajan, 1977). On the other hand, the increased stability of cross-linked agarose in 2 M guanidine HCl gives the chance to use higher flow rates and keep the separation time within reasonable limits.

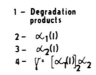

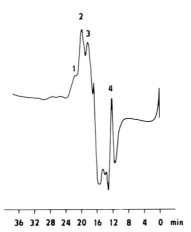

Fig. 4. Separation of polypeptide chains present in collagen type I preparation. 500 x 8 m Separon HEMA-Glc column eluted with 0.05 M Tris HCl (2 M urea) at 1.5 ml/min. Peaks of intermediate mobility between α and γ are (according to poly-acrylamide gel electrophoresis) β fractions (dimers of non-specified α-chains).

One of the great advantages of this procedure is the very high recovery of pepsin solubilized collagen (92-100% of deffated material as revealed by hydroxyproline balance studies). This is in a strong contradiction to the multiple step precipitation procedures which may lead to recoveries as low as 20% of the originally present hydroxyproline posi-tive material.

As indicated above, the two subsequent Bio-Gel A-1.5 m separations or the separation on Bio-Gel A 5 m and Sepharose CL 6B, can be replaced by fraction precipitation: By this method collagen type III including the portion bonded with non-reducible cross-links can be isolated in reasonably pure form (Chandrarajan and Klein, 1980).

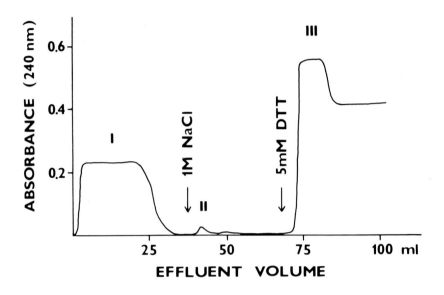

Fig. 5. Stepwise elution pattern of reduced and denatured pepsin-treated calf skin collagen from thiol-Sepharose column. The bulk of collagen does not bind is the column; further fractions are eluted with 1 M NaCl and 5 mM dithiothreitol.

    The chromatographic separations described can be classified as the conventional ones. For the separation of type I and III collagens by high-performance column liquid chromatography Separon HEMA-Glc (Laboratory Inst. Works, Prague) packing can be used. Elution is done isocratically with 0.5 M Tris- 2 M urea. The method offers a complete separation of $\alpha_1(I)\alpha_2$, $\alpha_1(III)$, $[\alpha_1(I)]_2\alpha_2$ and $[\alpha_1(III)]_3$ polypeptide chains (Macek et al., 1980) and lasts less than thirty minutes (Fig. 4).

    An effective separation of type I and III collagen can be achieved by covalent chromatography on thiol activated Sepharose 4B (Sykes, 1976). The non-specifically bound material is eluted with the starting buffer made 1 M with respect to NaCl. When absorbance has come back to zero, the buffer is supplemented with dithiothreitol (5 mM) and elution

is carried out until the absorbance of the eluate starts to
rise. At this moment elution is discontinued and the column
left for 40 min to release the bound material (Fig. 5).

Separation behaviour of collagen type II and related
materials

When papain treated cartilage collagen is subjected to
CM cellulose chromatography using a two chambered gradient
(0.06-0.05 M lithium acetate adjusted to pH 4.8, 6 M with
respect to urea) two peaks are observed in the chromatographic pattern. Of these the second peak is clearly not the
α_2 polypeptide chain as it behaves differently upon polyacrylamide gel electrophoresis. The osteoarthrotic collagen
reveals even four peaks. The differences in chromatographic
behaviour of individual α-polypeptide chains have been
ascribed to changed hydroxylation of osteoarthrotic type II
collagen (Fukae et al., 1975) and to altered glycosylation.

More recently, however, it was described that human
hyaline cartilages contains three minor collagenous proteins
different form the α_1(II) chain. These can be separated
(in denatured form) on CM cellulose (Burgeson and Hollister,
1979).

Separation of collagen III and IV

The necessity for separation collagen type III and type
IV arose from their simultaneous occurence in aortic wall.
Similary as with other insoluble collagen species, limited
proteolysis is the necessary step in analysing the above
naturally occurring collagen mixtures.

The peptic digest of aortic collagen (after complex
purification by precipitation with 20 and 15% sodium chloride)
can be separated on 8% agarose (Bio-Gel A-1.5 m, Trelstad,
1974). The γ fraction obtained in this way can be fractionated by CM cellulose chromatography into type IV and
III collagen. The method of separation on CM cellulose is
that of Piez et al. (1963). Incomplete separation can be
also achieved by direct CM cellulose chromatography without
preliminary Bio-Gel A-1.5 m separation.

Basement membranes collagens

Many controversial findings concerning the structure of type IV collagen have resulted from the use of pepsin for its extraction. This procedure degrades namely noncollagenous proteins and renders interstitial collagens (types I - III) soluble. Although the native triple helix of most collagen types is resistant to the action of pepsin there are some limitations of this method - nonhelical regions such as telopeptides, procollagen peptides and some sites within helical region in some collagens are not resistant to the action of pepsin. Some authors using single pepsin digestion have reported therefore a heterogenous mixture of type IV collagen fragments ranging after reduction of disulphide bonds from approximately 50 000 - 140 000 in rel. mol. mass. Molecular sieve and ion-exchange chromatography lead to a separation of alpha 1(IV) and alpha 2(IV) chains from other fragments.

Some years ago another basement membrane collagen was isolated, which has been termed "AB collagen". There is now sufficiently good evidence to categorize AB collagen as type V and to assign to this type three different chains, B, A, and C, to be designated as $\alpha1(V)$, $\alpha2(V)$ and $\alpha3(V)$, respectively. The molecular organization of type V collagen remains unclear. Other molecular species are identified by the value of their relative molecular mass only (Burgeson et al., 1976; Chung et al., 1976; Kresina and Miller, 1979; Rhodes and miller, 1978; Daniels and Chu, 1975; Timpl et al., 1978; Hudson and Spiro, 1972; Sato and Spiro, 1976).

One of the fundamental procedures worked out for the separation of A and B collagens as well as the 55 000 relative molecular mass fraction is that of Chung et al. (1976).

The material (large vessel walls, intima) after limited peptic digestion is removed collagen type I and III by the salting out method. Collagenous material remaining in the high salt concentration solution offers practically a single peak upon Sepharose 4B chromatography (Fig. 6A). After reduction with 2-mercaptoethanol the agarose pattern is changed as shown in Fig. 6B. The dominant peak here has a relative molecular mass of 55 000 and can be chromatographed on CM-cellulose in the position of type III collagen. Elution is carried out with a 0-0.12 M NaCl gradient superimposed

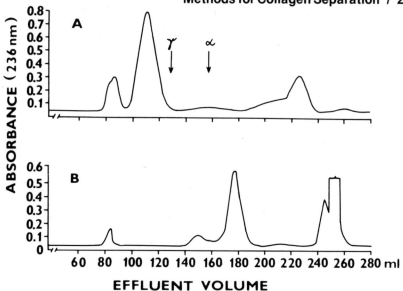

Fig. 6A. Sepharose 4B elution profile of the collagen-like protein isolated of human aortic intima.
Fig. 6B. Rechromatography of the major high molecular weight fraction (eluted at 110 ml in A) following reduction with 2-mercaptoethanol. The column was equilibrated and eluted at a flow rate of 10 ml/hr with 2.0 M guanidine-HCl pH 7.5 (0.05 M Tris). Arrows indicate the elution position of γ-components and α chains.

over the starting buffer. When skin collagen is subjected to the same procedure as described above for large vessel wall collagen, analogous profile is obtained. CM-cellulose chromatography of the same material results into two incompletely separated peaks corresponding to type A and B collagens as revealed by futher analyses.

Another strategy for the isolation and separation of A and B collagens was introduced by Bentz et al. (1978). This approach involves two separations on DEAE-cellulose with a gel chromatography inserted inbetween these two and belongs into the category of multidimensional separations. The bulk of collagenous material is removed from the mixture of A and B chains in the first DEAE-cellulose run while in the subsequent step the individual A and B chains are separated (Bentz et al., 1978) (collagen from amniotic-chorionic mem-

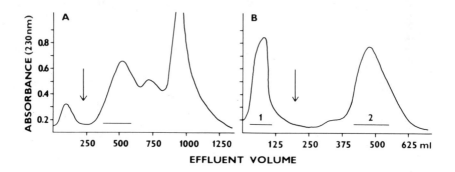

Fig. 7. DEAE-cellulose chromatography of native placental collagen. (A) DEAE-cellulose column (2.5 x 11 cm) was equilibrated at 42°C in 0.025 M Tris-HCl, 4 M urea, pH 8.6. Chromatography of the collagen fraction precipitated between 2.5 and 4.0 M NaCl. The peak containing A and B chains is marked by a bar. (B) Separation of the A and B chains by rechromatography on DEAE-cellulose. The start of the linear gradient of 0-0.1 M NaCl in a total volume of 1000 ml buffer is marked by arrows.

brane). In the first DEAE-cellulose chromatography the A and B collagens as well as other collagenous material are chromatographed in the native state at 15°C (Fig. 7AB). Next, polymers are removed from the isolated fraction of mixed A+B chains by Bio-Gel A-1.5 m chromatography. Separation of A and B collagen chains is carried out in the second DEAE-cellulose chromatographic step. Here, collagen is denatured prior the separation and a linear gradient of 0-0.1 M NaCl superimposed over the starting buffer is used for elution.

Alternatively CM-cellulose chromatography can replace the second DEAE-cellulose procedure (von der Mark and von der

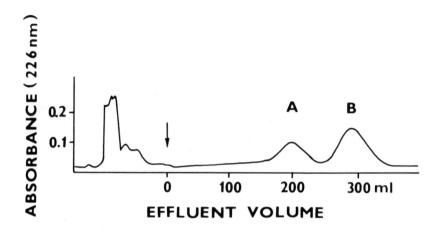

Fig. 8. Separation of A and B chains by CM-cellulose chromatography. A,B-collagen was denatured and applied to CM-cellulose column (1.5 x 12 cm) at 42°C, equilibrated in 0.04 M sodium acetate, 6 M urea (pH 4.8). Elution was achieved by a linear gradient between 0-0.12 M NaCl over 600 ml.

Mark, 1979). Separation is achieved by a linear gradient of 0-0.12 M NaCl (Fig. 8).

CM-cellulose can be used also for a partial separation of pepsin solubilized synovial membrane A, B, C and D collagens that can be isolated by precipitation and dialysis against 4 M NaCl after other collagenous materials have been removed. The precipitate obtained in this way shows three bands in polyacrylamide gel electrophoresis. Incomplete chromatographic separation of these components could be achieved on a CM-cellulose column using gradient elution (0-1.0 M NaCl).

Rhodes and Miller (1978) worked out a method for separating A and B collagens by phosphocellulose chromatography.

Elution is done with a linear NaCl gradient in the range 0.0-0.2 M (in starting buffer) and with denatured collagen samples.

Besides the protein with rel. mol. mass 55 000 and the A, B and perhaps C collagens, even more complex mixtures of basement membrane collagens can be recovered after limited proteolysis of placental mince (Kresine et al., 1979). In the first step A and B chains are removed from the proteolytic digest (Rhodes and Miller, 1978) by dializing the 0.1 M NaCl-0.05 M Tris pH 7.4 solution of the pepsin digest versus a large volume of 0.02 M NaCl containing 2M urea (0.01 M Tris pH 8.6). During this step a precipitate consisting of collagens composed of the A and B chains is formed. The supernatant solution contains futher collagenous material that can be separated as follows.

In the first step the material is subjected to CM-cellulose chromatography using gradient elution at $8^{O}C$ (Fig. 9). Collagen, recovered from the CM-cellulose step, is then rechromatographed on Bio-Gel A-5 m. The sample is denatured by warming and applied to a column that is eluted with 2 M guanidine hydroxychloride. Before further treatment individual fractions are desalted on a Bio-Gel P-2 column using 0.1 M acetic acid as mobile phase. Besides α^i and γ components a collagenous fraction of 50 000 rel. mol. mass is recovered (50K component).

The high molecular weight component (γ) is desalted subjected to reduction and alkylation, returned to the above Bio-Gel column and treated in the same way as the whole mixture. The position of α-chains (95 000) as well as 80 K and 40 K components, representing components of rel. mol. mass 80 000 and 40 000 respectively, can be traced in the elution profile. The rel. mol. mass of another component (C') is about 120 000.

The α-chain sized component obtained during the agarose separation of the crude mixture can be subjected to CM-cellulose separation under denaturing conditions.

The 50 000 rel. mol. mass fraction from the Bio-Gel chromatography (50 K fraction) when subjected to rechromatography on CM-cellulose under the same conditions as above, reveals a heterogenous collection of polypeptide fragments containing two major fractions, namely 50 K_1 and 50 K_2.

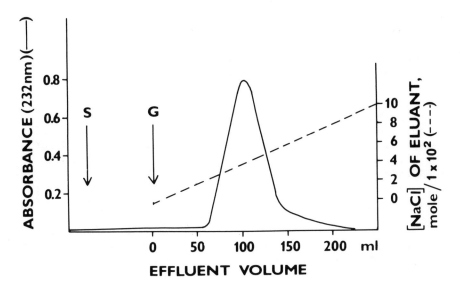

Fig. 9. CM-cellulose chromatography of collagen containing the C and D chains under nondenaturing conditions. The column was operated at 8°C and eluted at a flow rate of 100 ml/h by means of a linear gradient of 0-0.4 M NaCl in 0.04 M sodium acetate pH 4.8 (2 M with respect to urea) over total volume 1 1. The letter S denotes the point of sample application, and G indicates initiation of gradient.

It has to be noted that under conditions used here for CM-cellulose chromatography native types of I and III collagens as well as A and B chains are much more retained on the column and could not be visualized within the chromatographic profiles shown.

The so called C and D chains can be obtained also from glomerular basement membrane after pepsin treatment and isolated as a combined peak by Bio-Gel A 5 m chromatography. The third peak emerging from this separation can be resolved on CM-cellulose into C and D chains. Other fragments like the 15K protein can be obtained as well (Dixit and Kang, 1979, 1980; Dixit, 1979). Using Bio-Gel A-5 m and A-1.5 m, in combination with CM-cellulose it is possible to visualize the

D-1 and 75 K components (Dixit, 1980) and to separate C-1, D-1 and 75 K components side-by-side.

Bailey and coworkers (1979) identified another basement membrane collagen (besides the A and B chains) that normally coprecipitates with type I of pepsin digests of human placenta. Further characterization of this category of collagen polypeptides can be done on CM-cellulose.

The heterogeneity of basement membrane collagens can be further demonstrated by Bio-Gel A-5 m chromatography of material synthesized by Descement membrane cells in culture. Here a collagenous fraction of rel. mol. mass 155 000 can be observed (larger than that reported in cultures of lens cells and similar to procollagen peptidic chains of parietal yolk sac).

Two components categorized among basement membrane collagens were isolated from anterior lans capsule (Dixit, 1978). The second peak when subjected to reduction and carboxy-methylation and finally to gel permeation chromatography gives a complex pattern with main fractions of 110 000 and 50 000 rel. mol. mass.

High molecular weight material resembling pro-collagen chains was isolated also from tumor basement membrane (EHS sarcoma) (Timpl et al., 1978). Chromatography of this material can be done frist on DEAE-cellulose column under denaturation conditions with 0-0.3 M NaCl gradient superimposed over the starting buffer. The unretained peak contains $\sim$ 70% of total hydroxyproline applied to the column. The second fraction contained 20-30% of hydroxyproline while the rest was rather poor in this amino acid. Rechromatography of tumor basement membrane collagen on CM-cellulose column with gradient elution 0-0.2 M NaCl yielded the profile shown in Fig. 10. Further characterization of this chromatographically homogenous material by polyacrylamide gel electrophoresis indicated the presence of two types of polypeptide chains occuring in the pro-α chain region, i.e. with a mobility between α and β chains. These are not indentical with pro-α chains of normal basement membrane collagen.

Very recently (Risteli et al., 1980) a new collagenous protein (fraction) called 7S collagen was isolated from a mouse tumor basement membrane as well as from other sources used for the isolation of basement membrane collagens. This

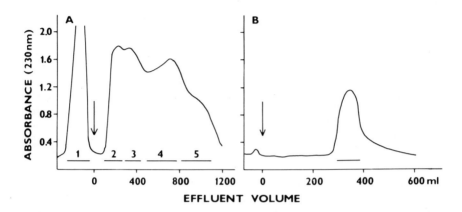

Fig. 10. Chromatography of tumor basement membrane proteins
first on DEAE-cellulose (A) then on CM-cellulose (B). (A)
DEAE-cellulose was equilibrated in 2 M urea, 0.05 M Tris-
HCl, pH 8.6 (column 2.5 x 20 cm). Protein fractions were
eluted with a linear gradient of 0-0.3 M NaCl in a volume of
1600 ml. The arrow denotes the start of the gradient. (B)
Rechromatography of tumor basement membrane collagen on CM-
cellulose in 8 M urea, 0.01 M sodium acetate, pH 4.8. The
collagenous material obtained after chromatography on DEAE-
cellulose (A, pool 1) was applied to a CM-cellulose column
(2.5 x 20 cm) and eluted with a linear gradient of 0-0.2 M
NaCl in a volume of 800 ml. The fractions containing tumor
basement membrane collagen are indicated by a horizontal bar
in the diagram. The arrow denotes the start of the gradient.

protein is susceptible to a two step chromatographic separation: first it is separated from the bulk of other proteins
by passing through a Bio-Gel A-5 m column followed by further
purification on CM-cellulose. Gradient of 0-0.2 M NaCl over
the starting buffer is used to elute the material from the
ion exchange column. It has to be stressed that preliminary
purification of the crude material on a DEAE-cellulose column
is necessary in this case.

Chromatographic behavior of collagen precursors

   The collagen precursor fraction is expected to contain
molecules with several size precursor chains; one with amino
extension 15 000 rel. molecular mass (pM α-chain), another with
a carboxy extension 3 500 rel. mol. mass, pC α-chain) and
one with both extensions (pro-α chain).

   The mixtures actually obtained are usually complex and
the interpretation of chromatographic data is usualy difficult (Davidson et al., 1975). Procollagen preparations
extracted from bone, purified by a complex procedure, can be
applied to a DEAE-cellulose column. Elution is done iso-
cratically at the beginning followed by a linear gradient
from 0-0.2 M NaCl. Peaks designed as A and B (not to be
confused with A and B of basement membrane collagens) contain
α_1 and α_2 chains only as revealed by subsequent polyacrylamide gel electrophoresis. The reason for the different
chromatographic behaviour of these fractions was not elucidated. Peak C while offering a complex polyacrylamide gel
pattern before reduction yields pro-α_1 and pro-α_2 besides
a low molecular weight peptide after reduction. Finally,
peak D (composed of material that hardly penetrated 5% polyacrylamide gel) when reduced offered pro-α_1 and pro-α_2 chains
as well. The complexity of the separation pattern before
reduction is obviously caused by interchain disulphide
bridges in the propeptide region.

   An alternative to DEAE-cellulose separation of collagen
precursors has been worked out by Smith et al., 1974. The
main difference here is the increased proportion of urea
(8 M) in the eluting buffer. Under such circumstances all
precursor molecules elute as a single peak.

   Denatured type I rat skin collagen precursors can be
fractionated futher on CM-cellulose. The pooled precursor
fraction (collagen type I from the DEAE cellulose chromatography) is transferred to a CM-cellulose column and eluted
with a linear gradient from 0 to 70 mM NaCl. At least six
major components are separated. The first eluting fraction
was identified as pN α_1, the second was a fraction containing two proteins - one undistinguishable from α_1 chain,
the other with molecular mass 145 000 (most likely pro-α_1).
The third peak according to polyacrylamide gel chromatography and CNBr peptide pattern is most likely pro-α_1, the

fourth (identification based on the same criteria) was pC α_1 precursor. The other two peaks contained only α_2 CNBr peptides indicating thus their relation to the α_2 chain. The first of these is split into two zones upon polyacrylamide gel electrophoresis, the α_2 chain and a precursor of rel. mol. mass 115 000. The other peak (last on CM-cellulose pattern) contained two zones corresponding to rel. mol. mass 130 000 and 140 000. It has been concluded that all the peptides with molecular mass higher than 100 000 represent three different precursors of $\alpha_2(I)$ collagen chain.

For the separation of $\alpha(II)$ procollagen polypeptides, pro(αII) and $[pro(\alpha II)]_3$ chains, both ion exchange chromatography and gel permeation chromatography can be used (Uitto et al., 1977).

In both cases the recoveries are almost quantitative and both methods can be used for preparative as well as analytical purposes.

An advanced procedure for the purification of procollagen type II by covalent chromatography on activated thiol Sepharose 4 B was reported by Angermann and Barrach (1979). The procedure runs as follows: purified procollagen is added to thiol Sepharose 4B, and after completion of the reaction the suspension is poured into a chromatographic column. Unbound collagen is eluted and the contaminating material is removed in a subsequent wash. The eluting buffer is then made 5 mM with respect to dithiothreitol and introduced into the column. When the dithiothreitol containing buffer starts to leave the column (as indicated by the rise of absorptivity at 240 nm) the flow is interrupted for a period sufficient to permit reduction of the material bound to the column. Then, continuing the elution, purified procollagen type II is eluted. The method was used for the purification of collagen from rat chondrosarcoma.

An even more complex (multi dimensional) chromatography has been elaborated for the type III collagen precursor chains, that can be extracted from skin by neutral salt solutions. The procollagen polypeptides are accumulated by fraction precipitation (30% ammonium sulfate) and finally purified by passing through a DEAE-cellulose column.

The component polypeptide chains of type III procollagen (proα$_1$(III) and pα$_1$(III)) differing in the extension attachment can be isolated by CM-cellulose chromatography similarly as type I collagen precursors, Bellamy and Bornstein, 1971 (see also Piez et al., 1963).

The fraction recovered in the α$_2$ position upon CM-cellulose separation (containing procollagenous material) can be rechromatographed on an Bio-Gel A-5 m column, where pro αIII polypeptide chain has a slightly higher mobility than α$_2$, because of its higher relative molecular mass. After limited peptic proteolysis normal α$_1$(III) is recovered as expected.

Separation of complex collagen mixtures avoiding limited proteolysis

Guilaume et al., 1978 have succeded in almost complete solubilization of insoluble collagen by using 1% sodium dodecyl sulfate (SDS) extraction combined with β-mercaptoethanol reduction. After the 1% SDS extraction of the tissue (solubilizing one part of the collagenous material) there remains an insoluble fraction still containing hydroxyproline. This very insoluble fraction when subjected to reduction and alkylation is also obtained under a soluble form.

The 1% SDS extracts are in avarage 80% of the total collagen and SDS + β-mercaptoethanol treatment brings another 17% of the total collagen into solution.

The extracts can be submitted to Bio-Gel A-50 m chromatography to get some information about the molecular species in the solution. Chromatography of the 1% SDS extractable fraction reveals the presence of a very large molecular weight fraction (Fig. 11) which emerges from the column with the void volume. When the course of separation is controlled by polyacrylamide gel electrophoresis, this fraction does not penetrate the gel. After β-mercaptoethanol treatment this very large rel. molecular mass fraction gives an acrylamide gel pattern consistent with the presence of type I procollagen.

Peak 2 contains several γ-polymers. After β-mercaptoethanol reduction this fraction yields together with larger molecules a band whose electrophoretic behaviour is consis-

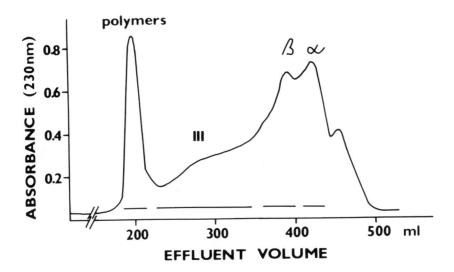

Fig. 11. Bio-Gel A-50 m (2% agarose) chromatography of the fraction extracted by 1% SDS. Elution was done with a sodium phosphate buffer pH 7.4 containing 1% SDS (90 x 2.5 cm column).

tent with that of α_1(III) chain. Peaks 3 and 4 represent β and α components respectively. The electrophoretic composition of the fraction which is only solubilized after reduction with β-mercaptoethanol is complex, predominantly with γ-components and non-collagen fractions.

Separation of collagen mixtures by zone precipitation chromatography

Besides chromatography, fraction precipitation appears the most widely used method for the isolation of collagen polypeptide chains. This method, however, can be also adopted by chromatography with a pronounced effect both in separation efficiency and separation time,(Ehrlich, 1979). A step-wise sodium chloride gradient is used to redissolve and precipitate collagens from the interbead space of a molecular sieve. Fundamental to zone precipitation is the fact that protein molecules are too big to enter the inter-

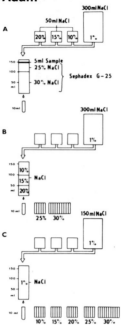

Fig. 12. A schematic view of Zone Precipitation Chromatography. All the salt solutions and sample are in 50 mM Tris-
HCl, pH 7.5 buffer. (A) A sample of 5 ml in buffered 1% NaCl
is layered on top of the column. The column is equilibrated
in buffered 30% NaCl (100 ml) followed by 25% NaCl (50 ml).
Separate 50 ml volumes of 20% NaCl, 15% NaCl, 10% NaCl and
300 ml of 1% NaCl are prepared and stand ready for application to the column. (B) 50 ml of the column elution is
collected in 12 ml fractions. First, 50 ml of the 20% NaCl
solution was applied followed by 50 ml of 15% NaCl solution
and then 50 ml of 10% NaCl solution. The 300 ml of 1% NaCl
solution stands ready for application. (C) 300 ml of the
column elution is collected in 12 ml fractions. 150 ml of
the 1% NaCl solution passes through the column and 150 ml is
left to be applied to the column. The optical density of
each fraction is read at 230 nm along with its conductivity.

bead space. They in fact move faster than the mobile phase
which penetrates the bead and has a longer distance to
traverse. When the protein in the solution outruns the
precipitant concentration where it is soluble, it occurs
finally at a higher salt concentration at which it precipitates from the solution. The solvent concentration, however,

after some time drops down. As a matter of fact it becomes so low that the precipitated protein goes back into solution. Since the precipitate is very fine, dissolution proceeds at a high rate. Finally the protein is eluted at the concentration which is characteristic for its dissolution. It is worth stressing that according to SDS-polyacrylamide gel electrophoresis type I collagen is represented here by three species which very likely reflects the fact that pepsin treatment produces heterogenous population of collagen type I molecules.

In practice tha column is partly equilibrated in 30% and partly in 25% NaCl (Fig. 12). The sample is applied and the column eluted with equal volumes of 20%, 15% and 10% saline. The eluate is collected in a fraction collector and the final wash of the column is done with 1% saline. The result of the separation is seen in Fig. 12. By this method it is possible to separate AB collagen, type I, type II and type III collagens side by side. The NaCl gradient can be replaced by ammonium sulphate with good results.

ELECTROPHORETIC SEPARATIONS

Conventional electrophoresis of collagen on polyacrylamide gel

As it has been demonstrated by Furthmayr and Timpl (1971) collagen peptides as well as intact α-chains exhibit a considerably lower electrophoretic mobility on SDS-polyacrylamide gels when compared to globular proteins of similar molecular weight. Another intresting feature is the separation of $\alpha_1(I)$ and $\alpha_2(I)$ polypeptide chains. The main reason for the special behavior of the collagen peptides in SDS-polyacrylamide gel electrophoresis seems to be a certain rigidity of the polypeptide structure even in the denatured state. It was shown that the restriction of mobility in the random coil conformation is due to the presence of imino acid residues that constitute a considerable portion of the collagen molecule. The higher mobility of the α_2 chain can probably be explained by its less rigid structure as reflected by lower denaturation temperature.

It can be excluded that a smaller negative change of collagenous proteins as compared to other protein categories is the reason for the atypical behavior during SDS-polyacryl-

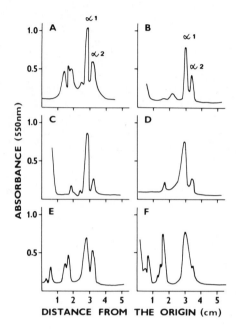

Fig. 13. Electrophoretic separation of collagen components.
The samples are derived from salt-fractionated material.
A, 1.5 M NaCl; B, 2.2 M NaCl; C, 2.4 M NaCl; D, 4.2 M NaCl;
E, type I collagen from rat skin; F, type II collagen from
rat chondrosarcoma.

amide gel electrophoresis. If it were true, then succinylated
or methylated collagens should exhibit a very different
electrophoretic behavior; in case of methylated collagen
the mobility should be lower than that of the native protein.
Just the opposite is, however, true. Also differences in the
amount of bound SDS can be exluded as the reason of the
anomalous behavior of collagen proteins. Besides others, the
differences between electrophoretic mobility of the $\alpha_1(I)$ and
$\alpha_2(I)$ chains are preserved even in the absence of SDS.

The diagnostic value of conventional SDS polyacrylamide
gel electrophoresis (7% gel) can be demonstrated best on
the profiles obtained with collagen fractions precipitable
at different NaCl concentration (Fig. 13, Moro and Smith,
1977).

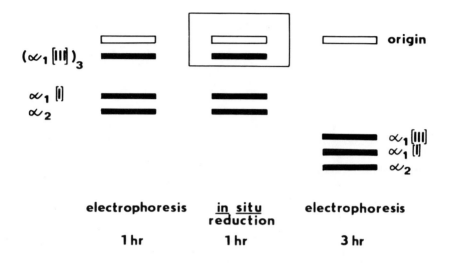

$(\alpha_1[III])_3$

$\alpha_1[I]$
α_2

origin

$\alpha_1[III]$
$\alpha_1[I]$
α_2

electrophoresis   **in situ**   **electrophoresis**
reduction

1 hr   **1 hr**   **3 hr**

Fig. 14. Principles of interrupted electrophoresis

Separation of collagen type I and III based on delayed reduction

By interrupting polyacrylamide gel electrophoresis (either in slabs or rods) about one hour after the collagen sample has been applied with concommittant reduction of collagen type III disulphide bonds in situ allows a complete separation of all three collagen α-chain species involved. At the time of reduction, $[\alpha_1(III)]_3$ chains have scarcely entered the gel, while $\alpha_1(I)$ and α_2 have travelled a certain distance. When the current is switched on again, the depolymerized $\alpha_1(III)$ chain penetrates the gel and starts to travel with some delay allowing thus a complete differentiation from $\alpha_1(I)$ and $\alpha_2(I)$ (Fig. 14). Instead of 6% slab gels (Sykes et al., 1976), rods can be used as well (Shuttleworth et al., 1978).

Separation of collagen type I and III based on CNBr cleavage

For the separation of collagen type I and III in small skin samples (tissue biopsies) SDS-polyacrylamide electrophoretic pattern of the CNBr peptides was used by Weber et al. (1977). 10 x 0.5 cm gels of 12% polyacrylamide containing 2% SDS can be used. After removal from the gel tubes the gels are evaluted by densitometry (540 nm) of the Coomassie Brilliant Blue stain.

Most of the bands appearing in the CNBr peptide mixture are complex and consist of peptides derived from different collagen chains. On the other hand there are a few bands that consist purely from type I or type III collagen peptides that can be used for quantitation.

Separation of basement membrane collagens

A and B collagens isolated from chick embryos can be separated by discontinous slab gel electrophoresis. The method used is in principle that of Laemmli (1970). 5-10% gel are used (Von der Mark and von Mark, 1979).

The A and B chains obtained after pepsin solubilization of human chorionic or allantoic membrane are susceptible to this category of separations as well.

Electrophoretic behavior of collagen precursors

Generally saying because of distinct differences in rel. molecular mass between individual types of collagen precursors, collagen α chains and their polymers, polyacrylamide gel electrophoresis is widely applied for these separations.

Thus SDS slab gel electrophoresis is recommendable as a tool for elucidating the step-wise cleavage of N- and C-terminal extensions during type I procollagen conversion to type I collagen (Davidson et al., 1975).

As far as collagen type II precursors is concerned, polyacrylamide gel electrophoresis according to King and Laemmli (1971) in slab gels results in a single band of $[\text{pro }\alpha(II)]_3$ chain. The mobility of this zone is not distinguishible from of $[\text{pro }\alpha(I)]_3$ that could be isolated from embryonic tendon cells. When the protein is reduced with

2-mercaptoethanol prior to application to the gel, it migrates at about the same speed as pro α(I) chains of type I collagen precursor.

Electrophoretic separation of component chains of type III procollagen and type I procollagen can be done on 5% sodium dodecylsulfate acrylamide gels. The method of Furthamayer and Timpl (1971) is used for this purpose (see also Lenaers and Lapiere, 1975).

The method of Laemmli (1979) has been also exploited recently to the separation of type IV procollagen (Alitalo, 1980).

REFERENCES

Adam M, Deyl Z, Macek K (1979). Ways of collagen separation in pathologically altered tissue. J Chromatogr 162:163.
Alitalo K (1989). Eur J Biochem in press.
Angermann K, Barrach HJ (1979). Purification of procollagen type II by covalent chromatography with activated thiol-Sepharose 4B. Anal Biochem 94:253.
Bailey AJ, Sims TJ, Duance VC, Light ND (1979). Partial characterization of a second basement membrane collagen in human placenta. Evidence for the existence of two type IV collagen molecular. FEBS Lett 99:361.
Bellamy G, Bornstein P (1971). Evidence for procollagen, a biosynthetic precursor of collagen. Proc Natl Acad Sci USA 68:1138.
Bentz H, Bächinger HP, Glanville R, Kühn K (1978). Physical evidence for the assembly of A and B chains of human placental collagen in a single triple helix. Eur J Biochem 92:563.
Burgeson RE, ElAdli FA, Kaitila II, Hollister DW (1976). Fetal membrane collagen, identification of two new collagen alpha chains. Proc Natl Acad Sci 73:2579.
Burgeson RE, Hollister DW (1979). Collagen heterogeneity in human cartilage: identification of several new collagen chains. Biochem Biophys Res Commun 87:1124.
Chandrajan J, Klein L (1980). Chromatographic separation and quantification of type I and type III collagens. J Chromatogr 182:94.
Chung E, Rhodes RK, Miller EJ (1976). Isolation of three collagenous components of probable basement origin from several tissues. Biochem Biophys Res Commun 71:1167.

Daniels JR, Chu GH (1975). Basement membrane collagen of renal glomerulus. J Biol Chem 250:3531.

Davidson JM, McEneany LSG, Bornstein P (1975). Intermediates in the limited proteolytic conversion of procollagen to collagen. Biochemistry 14:5188.

Dixit SN (1978). Isolation and characterization of two collagenous components from anterior lens capsule. FEBS Lett 85:153.

Dixit SN (1979). Isolation and characterization of two α chain size collagenous polypeptide chains C and D from glomerular basement membrane. FEBS Lett 106:379.

Dixit SN (1980). Type IV collagens. Isolation and characterization of two structurally distinct collagen chains from bovine kidney cortices. Eur J Biochem 106:563.

Dixit SN, Kang AH (1979). Anterior lens capsule collagens: cyanogen bromide peptides of the C chain. Biochemistry 18:5686.

Dixit SN, Kang AH (1980). Basement membrane collagens. Cyanogen bromide peptides of the D chain from porcine kidney. Biochemistry 19:2692.

Ehrlich HP (1979). Zone precipitation chromatography: its use in the isolation of different collagen type. Prep Biochem 9:407.

Fukae M, Mechamic GL, Adamy L, Schwartz ER (1975). Chromatographically different type II collagens from human normal and osteoarthritic cartilage. Biochem Biophys Res Commun 67:1575.

Furthmayr H, Timpl R (1971). Characterization of collagen peptides by sodium dodecylsulfate-polyacrylamide electrophoresis. Anal Biochem 41:510.

Guilaume G, Szymanovicz G, Rondoux A, Borel JP (1978). A fractionation of insoluble rat skin collagen. Biomed 29:5.

Hall DL (1976). "The methodology of Connective Tissue". Joynson-Bruwers, Oxford.

Hudson BG and Spiro RG (1972). Studies on the native and reduced alkylated renal glomerular basement membrane. Solubility, subunit size and reaction with cyanogen bromide. J Biol Chem 247:4229.

Huszar G, Maiocco J, Naftolin F (1980). Monitoring of collagen and collagen fragments in chromatography of protein mixtures. Anal Biochem 105:424.

Klein L, Chandrarajan J (1977). Collagen degradation in rat skin but not in intestine during rapid growth: effect on collagen types I and III from skin. Proc Natl Acad Sci USA 74:1436.

Kresina TF, Miller EJ (1979). Isolation and characterization of basement membrane collagen from human placental tissue. Evidence for the presence of two genetically distinct collagen chains. Biochemistry 18:3089.

Laemmli UK (1970). Cleavage of structural proteins during the assembly of the head of bacteriophage T4. Nature 227: 680.

Lenaers A and Lapiere CM (1975). Type III procollagen and collagen in skin. Biochim Biophys Acta 400:121.

Macek K, Deyl Z, Čoupek J, Sanitrák J (1980). Separation of collagen type I and III by high-performance column liquid chromatography. J Chromatogr in press.

Moro L, Smith BD (1977). Identification of collagen $\alpha_1(I)$ trimer and normal type I collagen in a polyoma virus-induced mouse tumor. Arch Biochem Biophys 182:33.

Piez KA (1967). Molecular weight determination of random coil polypeptides from collagen by molecular sieve chromatography. Anal Biochem 26:305.

Piez KA, Eigner E, Lewis M (1963). The chromatographic separation and amino acid composition of the subunit of several collagens. Biochemistry 2:58.

Risteli J, Bächinger HP, Engel J, Furthmayr H (1980). 7-S collagen: characterization of an unusual basement membrane structure. Eur J Biochem 108:239.

Rhodes RK, Miller EJ (1978). Physicochemically characterization and molecular organization of the collagen A and B chains. Biochemistry 17:3442.

Sato T, Spiro RG (1976). Studies on the subunit composition of the renal glomerular basement membrane. J Biol Chem 251:4062.

Smith BD, Byers PH, Martin GR (1974). Production of procollagen by human fibroblasts in culture. Proc Natl Acad Sci USA 69:3260.

Shuttleworth CA, Ward JL, Hirschmann PN (1978). The presence of type III collagen in the developing tooth. Biochem Biophys Acta 535:348.

Stegeman H (1958). Mikrobestimmung von Hydroxyprolin mit chloramin-T und p-diemethylaminobenzaldehyd. Hoppe-Seyler's Z Physiol Chem 311:41.

Sykes BS (1976). The separation of two soft-tissue collagens by covalent chromatography. FEBS Lett 61:180.

Sykes B, Puddle B, Francis M, Smith R (1976). The estimation of two collagens from human dermis by interrupted gel electrophoresis. Biochem Biophys Res Commun 72:1472.

Timpl R, Martin GR, Bruckner P, Wick G, Wiedemann H (1978). Nature of the collagenous protein in a tumor basement membrane. Eur J Biochem 84:43.

Trelstad RL (1974). Human aorta collagens: evidence for three distinct species. Biochem Biophys Res Commun 57:717.

Uitto J, Hoffman HP, Prockop DJ (1977). Purification and partial characterization of the type II procollagen synthesized by embryonic cartilage cells. Arch Biochem Biophys 179:654.

Von der Mark H, Von der Mark K (1979). Isolation and characterization of collagen A and B chains from chick embryo. FEBS Lett 99:101.

Weber L, Meigel WN, Rauterberg J (1977). SDS-polyacryl-amide gel electrophoretic determination of type I and type III collagen in small skin sample. Arch Dermatol Res 258:251.

Connective Tissue Research:
Chemistry, Biology, and Physiology, Pages 45-62
© **1981 Alan R. Liss, Inc., 150 Fifth Avenue, New York, N.Y. 10011**

ELASTIN: MOLECULAR AND SUPRAMOLECULAR STRUCTURE

A.M. Tamburro

Istituto di Chimica Analitica-
Universita di Padova
Via Marzolo 1, 35100 Padova, Italy.

INTRODUCTION

Elastic tissue is an important constituent of a variety
of mammalian tissues. It is composed primarily of a rubber-
like protein, elastin, which is responsible for the long-
range extensibility and reversible deformability that charac-
terizes elastic tissue.

There is at present a lively controversy as to what are
the structural arrangements of elastin that can be compatible
with its physicochemical and mechanical properties.

Briefly, the major questions are the following:
i)   At the molecular level, does the protein chain exist as
     a random coil, or does it have a definite structure?
     Consequently, is the elasticity of the protein purely
     entropic or not?
ii) At the supramolecular level, is the protein amorphous or
     fibrous?

Apparently, the main disagreement seems to lie in the
conclusions drawn from electron microscope and thermoelastic
measurements, respectively. As a matter of fact, the latter
are almost compatible with the classical rubber theory by
which elasticity is described in terms of changes in conformational entropy of the elastomers, assumed to be an
amorphous three-dimensional network (Flory, 1969). On the
other hand, microscopists (Gotte, 1977); Cleary and Cliff,
1978) have repeatedly shown elastin to result from a composite assembly of filamentous entities, the ultimate com-

ponent possibly being a rope-like structure, each with an overall diameter of 3.5-4.0 nm, consisting of paired filaments each 1.5 nm in width.

In an attempt to overcome these apparent conflicts I will try to organize my presentation starting from analyzing the molecular structure of elastin and then correlating it to both supramolecular structure and elasticity. Finally, the structural aspects involved in the molecular pathology of such processes as atherosclerosis and aging will be briefly discussed.

MOLECULAR STRUCTURE

The most relevant studies have been performed using α-elastin, the soluble crosslinked derivative obtained from elastin by oxalic acid hydrolysis (Mammi et al. 1968; Mammi et al. 1970; Tamburro et al. 1977; Tamburro et al. 1978) and synthetic polypeptides containing the repeating sequences naturally occurring in elastin (Urry and Long, 1976). Whereas α-elastin in dilute aqueous solution at room temperature is essentially unordered (Fig. 1), this is no longer true in concentrated aqueous solution or in mixed organic solvents (Fig. 2, 3). Multiple conformational transitions occur under these conditions where structures such the α-helix and the so called β-bends are clearly detected. The presence of β-bend structures, firstly hypothesized by Urry, has also been revealed by NMR for the synthetic polypeptides (Urry and Long 1976). A sort of microheterogeneity of the unsoluble elastin in water was shown by NMR studies, indicating that in fibres swollen in water the chain motion is somewhat restricted as compared with that present in organic solvents (Ellis and Packer 1976, 1977; Torchia and Sullivan 1977).

Therefore, the contraddiction arises that the polypeptide chains have more motional freedom just where more secondary structure is present. However, at this point two remarks should be put forward:
i) the presence of hydrophobic bonds in elastin has been inferred from numerous studies (Gosline 1976). Therefore the organic solvents could probably act by disrupting intermolecular hydrophobic interactions and therefore enhancing chain mobility;

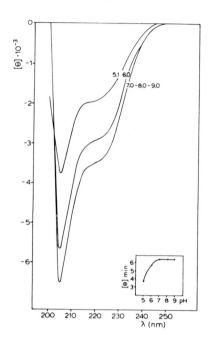

Fig. 1. CD spectra of α-elastin in 0.01 M Tris·HCl buffer at the indicated pH values. In the insert is reported the variation of the mean residue molecular ellipticity at the minimum of the shorter wavelengths negative band as a function of pH.

ii) the absence of a regular, periodic structure does not itself indicate a lack of rigidity. Actually, it could well be that some regions of elastin in water, although irregular, have restricted motional freedom.

In any case, being the chain flexible to allow conformational changes, the details of the bonds will be unimportant for large correlation distances. It is these large distances, greater than ∿ 50 Å, which are important in rubber elasticity (Deal and Edwards 1976). Bearing this in mind one can reasonably suggest that the molecular structure of elastin in water is essentially aperiodic with a fairly high degree of conformational flexibility. This is inferred from the multiple conformational transitions occurring when the solvent composition is changed and it does

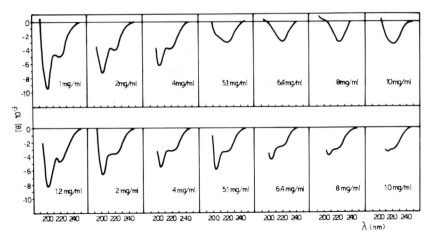

Fig. 2. CD spectra in aqueous solution (pH 7.4) of α-elastin in the absence (upper part) and in the presence (lower part) of $CaCl_2$ at the indicated protein concentrations. The molar ratio between $CaCl_2$ and α-elastin was $\sim 10^3$.

not appear as unexpected in wiew of the high amount of glycine residues present in this protein. This property of the protein can be easily related to such a labile struc- ture which changes on varying the solvent composition or in the presence of various solutes in order to produce a system of minimum free energy. A further example of the conforma- tional flexibility of this protein will be given in the last section of my presentation, where the structural changes induced in α-elastin interacting with lipids will be dis- cussed. A quite different picture, the so called fiblillar model, has been derived from studies on synthetic sequential polypeptides (Urry and Long 1976). Urry and coworkers studied the repeating polypeptides $(Val-Pro-Gly-Gly)_n$, $(Val-Pro-Gly-Val-Gly)_n$ and $(Ala-Pro-Gly-Val-Gly-Val)_n$ in chloroform, dimethylsulfoxide, methanol, trifluoroethanol and water. The possible conformations of the monomers were also examined by means of extensive conformational energy calculations (Urry and Long 1977). All of the repeat peptides were found to contain the β-bend or β-turn as a dominant conformational feature. In the organic solvents and in water only the β-turn is formed by the polytetrapeptide with the exception of elevated temperatures (above 50°C) in water where the dominant structure appears to be the cross-β-structure. The

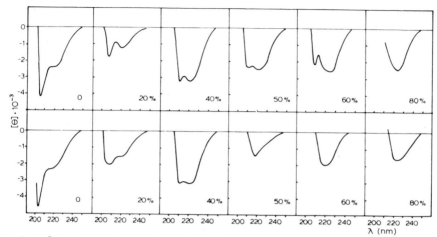

Fig. 3. CD spectra of α-elastin at room temperature in water-dioxane mixtures at the indicated percentages of the organic solvent in the absence (upper part) and in the presence (lower part) of $CaCl_2$ (1 mg/ml). The concentration of the protein was 1 mg/ml.

Gly-Val-Gly sequence which is common to both the pentamer and hexamer introduces a second conformational feature, called a γ-turn.

The pentameric subunits can form helical array referred to as β-spirals. The appearance of the overall structure is one of long spiralling ridges, alternatively hydrophobic and hydrophilic. However, it should be clearly understood that these structural features are neither rigid nor present under all circumstances. Significantly, in chloroform and in water above 50°C the cross-β-structure reappears at the expense of the γ-turn. The polyhexapeptide exhibits the same features as the polypentapeptide: here, however, there is, in addition, evidence for hydrogen bonding involving the NH of the last valine of one repeat and the valine CO of another. The result is a less mobile β-spiral. Differently from the polypentapeptide, the hydrophobic ridges of the polyhexapeptide β-spirals are discontinuous and disposed at angles of about 40°C to β-spiral axis, so that a ridge from one molecule can become interposed between two ridges of the associating molecule providing the appropriate properties for an interlocking role. These conformational features and

the suggestion of Gray et al. (1973) on the preference for
the α-helical conformation of the polyalanine sequences near
the cross-links were included in a three-component model.
The filamentous organization is constituted by three regions:
a) the cross-linking α-helical polyalanine segment; b) the
interlocking polyhexapeptide β-spiral; c) the dynamic,
elastomeric polypentapeptide β-spiral.

SUPRAMOLECULAR STRUCTURE

. A considerable amount of experimental evidence has been
obtained on the supramolecular structure of elastin by using
X-ray diffraction, light microscopes (Gotte 1976, 1977;
Serafini Fracassini et al. 1978; Cleary and Cliff 1978).
These experiments showed that elastin results from an assembly of rope-like structures each with an overall diameter of
3.5 or 4.0 nm containing paired filaments of indefinite
length. Each filament is about 1.5 nm in width and periodi-
cally linked longitudinally at a distance of 3.5-4.5 nm,
according to the degree of stretching. These results have
been correlated to those obtained at molecular level for
synthetic polypeptides in the following way: from the CPK
atomic model of the polyhexapeptide, the diameter of the
synthetic polymer is 1.5 nm, whereas the translation along
the spiral axis per β-turn was found to be 0.44 nm. The
X-ray diffraction data of elastin showed a diffuse ring at
0.44 nm both when the fibre was dry or swollen in dimethylsulfoxide (Gotte 1976, 1977). This ring could be accounted
for by the 0.44 nm translation per repeat along the spiral
axis of the chain. Such assignment has constituted the
basis for a new molecular explanation of the rubber-like
properties of elastin (Urry 1974; Gotte 1976). Accordingly,
the rubber-like behaviour of elastin was related to the
hydrated β-spiral segments occurring in the repeating penta-
and hexapeptide sequences. In terms of β-spiral, the hydrogen bonding between stacked β-bends would prevent extension
whereas hydration would allow disruption of these hydrogen
bonds and allow the bellows-like structure to extend. As
reported, the 0.44 nm repeat in dry elastin has been explained by the stacking of β-turns along the spiral. Addition of water results in a loss of the 0.44 nm ring: this
would correspond to the breaking of the hydrogen bonds
between turns of the spiral and the onset of elasticity.

However, two main arguments can be put forward against this proposal:

i) A diffuse ring at about 0.45 nm is compatible with almost proposable protein structure, especially when it is obtained on unoriented specimens.

ii) The disappearance of the ring in elastin swollen in water is of uncertain meaning since this is still present in elastin swollen in dimethylsulfoxide, a solvent which is thought to form stronger hydrogen bonds with protein functional groups than does water.

Finally, more recent studies using freeze-fracture electron microscopy (Pasquali Ronchetti et al. 1979) showed that unstretched elastin appears as a disordered granular material. A filamentous organization, consisting of filaments of about 5 nm across, only become visible after 180-200% of stretching.

INTERACTION WITH LIPIDS

The interaction between lipids and elastin seems to be strongly involved in processes such as atherogenesis and aging of elastic tissue. In an attempt to gain further insight into this problem we have studied, by circular dichroism spectroscopy, the conformational effects induced by the above mentioned compounds on α-elastin. For sake of comparison we investigated the modified protein obtained both from bovine ligamentum nuchae and from young and old human aortas.

The Fig. 4 shows the effect of sodium taurocholate on the conformation of α-elastins. At low taurocholate concentrations the CD spectra resembled those found for bovine α-elastin in organic solvents or at high protein concentration (Tamburro et al. 1977, 1978), and this was interpreted as arising, at least in part, from the β-bend conformation. Increasing the taurocholate concentration induced anomalous CD spectra of the proteins. In fact, the spectra were progressively shifted towards a unique negative band at about 217 nm with greatly enhanced optical activity, depending on the bile salt concentration. The enhancement of optical activity was similar to that found for liquid crystalline structures. From an analysis of the CD spectra we suggest that the major ordered arrangement of α-elastin consists of layers of β-structured polypeptide chains within

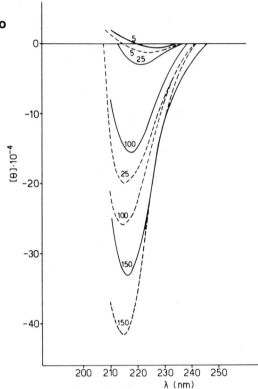

Fig. 4. CD spectra of α-elastins (0.02 mg/ml) in the presence of sodium taurocholate at the indicated concentrations
(mg/ml). 0.05M Tris-Cl buffer, pH 7.2 (- - -): human senile
and juvenile α-elastins; (———): bovine α-elastin.

the bile salt liquid crystal, producing a supramolecular
ordered array whose asimmetry affords the anomalous optical
activity. The observed trends are very similar for the
three proteins even if the human ones show more pronouced
band intensities. The next figures illustrate the effect
of unsaturated fatty acids.

We generally observe that the spectral features typical
of α-elastin, reflecting a predominantly aperiodic conformation, are deeply altered. As a matter of fact, multiple conformational variations are seen which depend on the nature
and concentration of the fatty acids and on the source of
α-elastin. For the bovine protein, as the concentration
of the fatty acids, here exemplified by linoleate (Fig. 5),

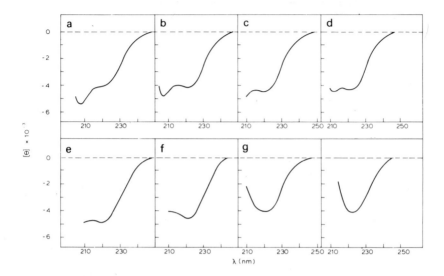

Fig. 5. CD spectra of α-elastin (0.02 mg/ml) in 0.05M sodium borate buffer. pH 10.0, in the presence of linoleate at different concentrations: (a)2; (b)3; (c)4; (d)5; (e)6; (f)7; (g)8; (h)30mM.

increased the amount of α-helical structure initially increased, then decreased and tended towards a new conformation characterized by a predominant negative band at ∿ 220 nm. The possibility exists that the new conformation observed on increasing the fatty acid concentration is, indeed, the β-bend structure. The Fig. 6 shows the effect of 25 mM oleate.

At this concentration of the fatty acid only the human senile protein is able to assume the β-conformation as judged by the negative band a 217 nm, while the other two proteins are in a partially α-helical structure.

In the case of human proteins the presence of the β-bend conformation was never evidentiated. In the presence of linoleate and palmitoleate (Figs. 7,8) the juvenile protein assumed only a partially helical conformation while the senile one showed also a β-like conformation at higher concentrations of the fatty acids.

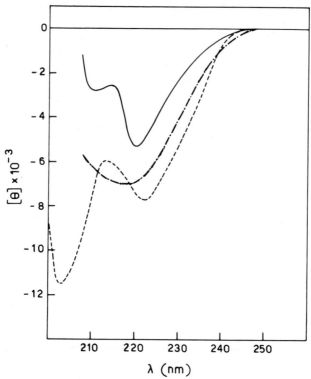

Fig. 6. CD spectra of α-elastins (0.3 mg/ml) in the presence of 25 mM oleate in 0.05 M borate buffer, pH 10.0. (——): bovine α-elastin; (- - -): human juvenile α-elastin; (- • -): human senile α-elastin.

A decrease in the α-helical structure was significantly favoured when both unsaturated fatty acids, at the highest concentration, were used, and sodium taurocholate was added to an aqueous solution of bovine α-elastin (Fig. 9). The Fig. 10 shows that similar behavior is also exhibited by the juvenile human protein. In these cases a predominant negative band appeared thourought at 215–217 nm, a wavelength typical of the amide n-π* transition associated with β-like structures.

All data presented can be summarized in the following scheme.

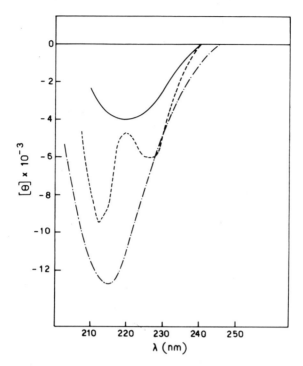

Fig. 7. CD spectra of α-elastins in the presence of 8 mM linoleate.
Solvent, concentrations and symbols as in Fig. 6.

Taurocholate at lower concentrations induces a β-bend structure and at higher concentrations a β-like structure in all proteins. The final conformation seems to be that derived from an inclusion of the β-structured α-elastin in some kind of liquid crystal.

On the other hand, the unsaturated fatty acids, when alone, are able to induce the β-structure only in the α-elastin from old human aortas, the conformational transition being stopped at the level of the α-helix for the juvenile protein and at the level of the β-bend for the bovine protein.

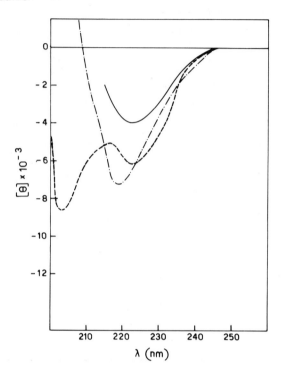

Fig. 8. CD spectra of α-elastins in the presence of 45 mM palmitoleate.
Solvent, concentrations and symbols as in Fig. 6.

CONCLUSIONS

   Keeping in mind all the reported data I believe that it is worth while making an effort in order to correlate the great deal of experimental conflicting results to the structure and the functional behaviour of elastin.

   First of all the discrepancy between the essentially unordered structure which turns out to be the most probable for elastin at the molecular level and the ordered organization shown by the same elastomer at the supramolecular level could be only apparent and not real since disorder at molecular scale does not necessarily mean disorder at the supramolecular scale. It would be possible to be dealing with fibres amorphous internally but in the same time associated

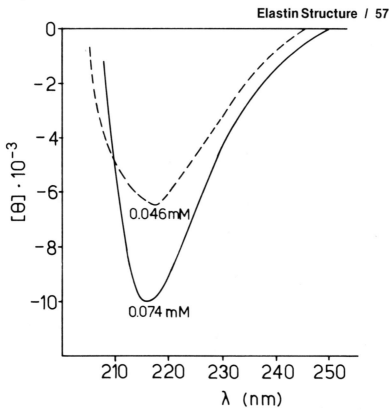

Fig. 9. CD spectra of bovine α-elastin in the presence of 45 mM oleate and 74 mM sodium taurocholate (——); and of 45 mM palmitoleate and 46 mM sodium taurocholate (- - -). Solvent: 0.05 M borate buffer, pH 10.1.

in some kind of regular arrangements. However, a more fruitful interpretation can be proposed.

Briefly, the following points should be appreciated:
i) All the known mechanical properties of elastin [particularly the presence of a glass transition (Kakivaya and Hoeve 1975; Gosline and French 1979)] are typical of amorphous, rubber-like polymers displaying "classical" elasticity, that is the enthalpy component of the retractive force is small and the entropy component is large.
ii) Chain mobility and conformational flexibility are features of water-swollen elastin (Torchia and Sullivan 1977; Ellis and Packer 1976, 1977; Tamburro et al. 1977, 1978; Guantieri et al. 1980). Obviously this does not

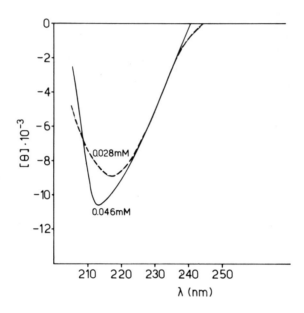

Fig. 10. CD spectra of human juvenile α-elastin in the presence of 45 mM oleate and 46 mM sodium taurocholate (——); and of 45 mM palmitoleate and 28 mM sodium taurocholate (- - -).
Solvent: 0.05 M borate buffer, pH 10.1

exclude the presence of transient and short-range structures, such as α-helices and β-bends, originated by small, dynamic clusters of non polar groups. This is quite compatible with the random-network model of rubber elasticity. Actually, randomness does not mean that all conformations are equally probable. To the contrary, the statistical theory is based on definite conformational states that have different probabilities depending on their energies. Simply, the conformations very rapidly switch over into one another. Accordingly, the organized structures proposed by Urry and coworkers for the synthetic polypeptides should be seen as local- ized and transient entities in the case of water-swollen elastin. This indicates that they are marginal as far

HUMAN SENILE α-ELASTIN

HUMAN JUVENILE α-ELASTIN

BOVINE α-ELASTIN

abbreviations: UFA, unsaturated fatty acids;
T, sodium taurocholate.

SCHEME: Conformational transitions of α-elastin.

as the elasticity is concerned and last but not least because these repeating sequences do not represent more than 15% of the tropoelastin aminoacid sequence.

iii) More ordered arrangements can arise in α-elastin and in the synthetic polypeptides when the pure aqueous environment is somewhat changed. It should be noted that the apparently unrelated changes such as the increase of temperature, the addition of organic solvents or lipids, the increase of protein concentration, are all amenable to a decreased activity of water, i.e. to a decreased effective concentration of water. Furthermore, the dominant structure is in any case the β-bend or a sort of β-like structure, possibly a cross-β-structure which could be easily derived from the β-bend. These are hydrogen-bonded, inelastic structures and it could well explain the plasticizing effect of water, that is the protein is elastic when swollen in water while it becomes brittle on dehydration. The disruption of the hydrogen bonds by water is needed for the recovery of the chain mobility and therefore of the elasticity. Parenthetically, this would also be the case of dimethylsulfoxide and in fact elastin is elastomeric when swollen in this solvent.

Turning to the supramolecular structure, as revealed by electron microscopy, I would suggest that the filamentous organization could, at least in part, arise from the final dehydration in the microscope. Stretching could also contribute. Conceivably, the molecular structure inside the dehydrated filaments may be again a β-like conformation: β-structured polypeptides are known to form fibrils (Gratzer et al. 1968).

iv) It is to be noted that the formation of a β-like structure seems to be deeply associated both to the interaction with the lipids and to the aging process. This has to be related to prior observations of Franzblau and coworkers (Jordan 1974; Mukherjee et al. 1976) that unsaturated fatty acids markedly decrease the tensile strength of fibres of elastin and greatly enhance the susceptibility of the protein to elastase. Furthermore, we have observed (Tamburro et al. 1980) that human senile elastin is more sensible to elastase than the juvenile protein.

Therefore, it seems that the same inelastic structure formed under a high lipid concentration would also be responsible for the breaks that occur in the polypeptide chain as part of the aging process. It is hoped that

these suggestions, admittedly speculative ones, will
stimulate further research on the molecular pathology
of elastin.

Cleary EG, Cliff WJ (1978). The substructure of elastin.
  Exp Mol Pathol 28:227.
Deam RT, Edwards FRS (1976). The theory of rubber elasticity.
  Phil Trans Roy Soc (London) 280:317.
Ellis GE, Packer KJ (1976). Nuclear spin relaxation studies
  of hydrated elastin. Biopolymers 15:813.
Ellis GE, Packer KJ (1977). Nuclear spin relaxation studies
  of elastin, II. A preliminary investigation of the effects
  of stretching and solvent composition on proton transverse
  relaxation. In Sandberg LB, Gray WR, Franzblau C (eds):
  "Elastin and Elastic Tissue". Adv Exp Med Biol 79:663.
  New York: Plenum Press.
Flory PJ (1969). "Statistical Mechanics of Chain Molecules".
  New York: Interscience.
Gosline JM (1976). The physical properties of elastic tissue.
  Int Rev Comm Tissue Res 7:211.
Gosline JM, French CJ (1979). Dynamic mechanical properties
  of elastin. Biopolymers 18:2091.
Gotte L (1976). Recent observations on the structure and
  composition of elastin. In Markham R, Horne RW (eds):
  "Structure-Function Relationships of Proteins". Amsterdam:
  Elsevier/North-Holland Biomedical Press, p 39.
Gotte L (1977). Recent observations on the structure and
  composition of elastin. In Sandberg LB, Gray WR, Franzblau
  C (eds): "Elastin and Elastic Tissue". Adv Exp Med Biol
  79:105. New York: Plenum Press.
Gratzer WB, Beaven GH, Rattle HW, Bradbury EM (1968). A
  conformational study of glucagon. Eur J Biochem 3:276.
Gray WR, Sandberg LB, Foster JA (1973). Molecular model for
  elastin structure and function. Nature 246:461.
Guantieri V, Tamburro AM, Daga-Gordini D (1980). Confor-
  mational changes induced in α-elastin by cholesterol,
  taurocholate and unsaturated fatty acids. Int J Biol
  Macromol 2:68.
Jordan RE, Hewitt N, Lewis W, Kagan H, Franzblau C (1974).
  Regulation of elastase-catalyzed hydrolysis of insoluble
  elastin by synthetic and naturally occurring hydrophobic
  ligands. Biochem 13:3497.
Kakivaya SR, Hoeve CAJ (1974). The glass point of elastin.
  Proc Nat Acad Sci USA 72:3505.

Mammi M, Gotte L, Pezzin G (1968). Evidence for order in the structure of α-elastin. Nature 220:371.

Mammi M, Gotte L, Pezzin G (1970). Comparison of soluble and native elastin conformations by far-ultraviolet circular dichroism. Nature 225:380.

Mukherjee DP, Kagan HM, Jordan RE, Franzblau C (1976). Effect of hydrophobic elastin ligands on the stress-strain properties of elastin fibers. Conn Tissue Res 4:177.

Pasquali-Ronchetti I, Formieri C, Baccarani-Contri M, Volpin D (1979). The ultrastructure of elastin revealed by freeze-fracture electron microscopy. Micron 10:89.

Serafini-fracassini A, Field JM, Hinnie J (1978). The primary filament of bovine elastin. J Ultrastruct Res 65:190.

Tamburro AM, Guantieri V, Daga-Gordini D, Abatangelo G (1977). Conformational transitions of α-elastin. Biochim Biophys Acta 492:370.

Tamburro AM, Guantieri V, Daga-Gordini D, Abatangelo G (1978). Concentration-dependent conformational transition of α-elastin in aqueous solution. J Biol Chem 253:2893.

Tamburro AM, Guantieri V, Daga-Gordini D (1980) unpublished observations.

Torchia DA, Sullivan CE (1977). A ^{13}C magnetic resonance study of embrionic chic aorta. In Sandberg LB, Gray WR, Franzblau C (eds): "Elastin and Elastic Tissue". Adv Exp Med Biol 79:655. New York: Plenum Press.

Urry DW (1974). Studies on the conformation and interactions of elastin. In "Arterial Mesenchyme and Arteriosclerosis". Adv Exp Med Biol 43:211. New York: Plenum Press.

Urry DW, Long MM (1976). Conformations of the repeat peptides of elastin in solution. CRC Crit Rev Biochem 4:1.

Urry DW, Long MM (1977). On the conformation, concervation and function of polymeric models of. elastin. In Sandberg LB, Gray WR, Franzblau C (eds): "Elastin and Elastic Tissue". Adv Exp Med Biol 79:685. New York: Plenum Press.

Connective Tissue Research:
Chemistry, Biology, and Physiology, Pages 63–71
© **1981 Alan R. Liss, Inc., 150 Fifth Avenue, New York, N.Y. 10011**

STRUCTURAL GLYCOPROTEINS AND OTHER CONNECTIVE TISSUE PROTEINS

John C. Anderson

Department of Medical Biochemistry, Medical School,
University of Manchester, Manchester, U.K.

The purpose of this article is to summarise the
important contributions made to our knowledge of this
subject since the last meeting when this field was reviewed
(Anderson, 1980).   This account will not include a
discussion of fibronectin or glycoproteins closely
associated with basement membranes, proteoglycans or
calcifiable matrices, since these will probably be dealt
with elsewhere in this volume.

Strictly speaking, we understand by the term structural
glycoprotein a macromolecule that is only solubilised by
extraction with guanidinium chloride or urea, usually after
prior removal of collagen.   However, release of a
glycoprotein from the matrix by treatment with bacterial
collagenase or extraction with a chaotropic agent may not
indicate a structural role since the glycoprotein may merely
be occluded between collagen fibrils.   It is intended in
this discussion to include other species that are secreted
by the cell.

Glycoproteins of connective tissues may be considered
in three groups: glycoproteins originating from plasma
(Mbuyi et al, 1980; Anderson, 1976); glycoprotein enzymes,
some concerned with collagen biosynthesis and maturation;
and thirdly, glycoproteins such as fibronectin and
microfibrillar protein, which have a structural or
morphogenetic role.

GLYCOPROTEIN ENZYMES

Prolyl hydroxylase consists of two α subunits (mol. wt. 64 000) and two β subunits (mol. wt. 60 000). Contrary to earlier reports it has now been shown that both subunits are glycoproteins and the monosaccharide content of each has been determined (Berg et al 1979). However, the α subunit binds to concanavalin A much more strongly than the β subunit does. Further evidence has now accrued establishing that the smaller prolyl hydroxylase subunit is easily extracted from tissues. Prolyl hydroxylase and an immunologically related smaller protein (cross-reacting protein, CRP) were extracted from young rabbit skin by mild methods and purified (Chichester et al, 1979). From half lives it was concluded that CRP is a precursor of active enzyme. A subsequent publication (Kao et al, 1980) reported that CRP (here defined as β subunit) is associated with the plasma membrane of L-929 fibroblasts, and there was a small concentration of CRP in the culture medium from tendon fibroblasts.

Miller and Varner (1979) extracted lysyl hydroxylase from fetal porcine skin using dilute tris buffer and showed that it consisted of subunits of mol. wts. 70 000 and 115 000. It appears that this lysyl hydroxylase differs from that of other species (chick and cow) which have a single subunit of 88 000.

The cleavage of procollagen to collagen monomer is thought to involve the action of at least two proteinases, one acting at the carboxyl terminal and the other acting at the amino terminal. Amino procollagen peptidase from embryonic chick tendon is a glycoprotein of mol. wt. 260 000, and requires Ca^{2+} for activity (Tuderman et al, 1978).

It now seems that an enzyme similar to, but not identical with cathepsin D, may be carboxyl procollagen peptidase. Such a glycoprotein enzyme, of mol. wt. 43 000 has been demonstrated in embryonic chick tendons and in tendon fibroblast cultures, and is able to effect the removal of C-terminal extension peptide from procollagen (Davidson et al, 1979).

No fresh evidence has emerged to elucidate the fate of the excised carboxyl and amino terminal procollagen peptides, which are both glycoproteins. Moczar et al (1979) have shown that aorta smooth muscle cells in culture secrete a glycoprotein of mol. wt. 36 000 (see later), which might correspond to carboxyl procollagen peptide.

Lysyl oxidase, unlike other enzymes concerned with post-translational modifications of collagen, is not extractable from tissues under mild conditions, but requires 4M-urea. Enzyme extracted from bovine aorta was resolved into four enzymatically active species (Kagan et al, 1979). Each had a subunit mol. wt. of 30 000, but aggregates of mol. wts. up to 10^6 could be formed.

A report at this meeting (Serafini-Fracassini et al, 1980) describes the characterisation of a self associating glycoprotein extracted from bovine ligamentum nuchae with 5M-guanidinium chloride containing reducing agents. This glycoprotein, of mol. wt. 21 000, demonstrated both amine oxidase activity and specific lysyl oxidase activity.

Extracellular appearance of intracellular enzymes is by no means restricted to those concerned with collagen biosynthesis and maturation. It is well known now that lysosomal exoglycosidases responsible for degradation of glycosaminoglycan chains are secreted from cells and that most of them are glycoproteins and contain a phosphohexosyl residue which is the recognition marker essential for pinocytosis (Kaplan et al, 1977).

PROPERTIES OF SOLUBLE GLYCOPROTEINS

A high mol. wt. (227 500) glycoprotein (LGP-I) has been shown to be the major constituent in the articular lubricating fluid from bovine synovial fluid (Swann et al, 1977). A second glycoprotein of mol. wt. 45 800 has now been isolated, and its composition determined (Swann and Mintz, 1979).

EXTRACTION AND PROPERTIES OF MATRIX-ASSOCIATED GLYCOPROTEINS

Randoux et al (1978) prepared a homogeneous glycoprotein (mol. wt. 16 000) from rabbit dermis by bacterial collagenase digestion and subsequent extraction of the residue with 8M-urea-mercaptoethanol, followed by purification on Sepharose 4B. Addition of this glycoprotein to human foreskin fibroblast cultures caused alterations in the incorporation of ^{14}C-proline into hydroxyproline.   At concentrations of less than 25 μg/ml there was a significant increase in collagen synthesis, while at concentrations above 50 μg/ml there was decreased incorporation into collagen.

Aalto et al (1979) isolated two glycoproteins (mol. wts. 59 000 and 71 000) from experimental rat granulation tissue. It was observed that these glycoproteins were able to inhibit collagen synthesis in embryonic tendon cells at concentrations down to 1 μM, so that their effect appears similar to that reported by Randoux et al (1978).

Gradient density ultracentifugation has been used by Bowness (1978) to compare the lipid binding ability of ^{125}I-labelled glycoproteins and albumin.   Glycoproteins were fractions A and G from puppy rib cartilage (Shipp and Bowness, 1975) and bovine aorta glycoprotein prepared by the procedure of Moczar et al (1977).   These associated with lipid or lipoprotein while albumin did not.   In addition, glycoproteins prepared from tissues that had not been delipidated contained a fraction already associated with lipid.   Glycoprotein-lipid binding was suggested to be one of the mechanisms involved in intercellular deposition of plasma lipoproteins in atherosclerosis.

It is appropriate at this point to examine in detail a recent report of an attempt to define aorta structural glycoprotein by analysis of all fractions extracted (Bach and Bentley, 1980).

Homogenised bovine aorta was first extracted sequentially with saline, sodium bicarbonate and EDTA which together removed a total of 10% of the dry weight of the tissue.   Polyacrylamide gel electrophoresis (PAGE) showed that these extracts contained a complex mixture of proteins. Most prominent were bands corresponding to haemoglobin, actin, albumin and an unknown protein of mol. wt. 24 000 (the latter two in saline extracts only).

The residue was then extracted with acetone and then nine times with 0.2mM-ATP - 0.2mM-ascorbate pH 7.5 at 4°. The latter removed a further 1.1% of the tissue dry weight. These aqueous extracts again appeared as complex mixtures on PAGE, showing a principal band corresponding in mobility

with actin, together with other bands of greater mobility.
Bands corresponding to molecular weights of 17 000, 31 000
and 43 000 were isolated by preparative electrophoresis and
analysed for amino acids. The latter protein contained
3-methyl histidine, a characteristic component of actin.

Three further extractions were made with 5M-guanidinium
chloride - 0.1%-EDTA - 0.05M-tris pH 8.5 at 4°, which removed
12% of the dry weight of the tissue. Again PAGE revealed
many bands in these extracts, but by preparative
electrophoresis and amino acid analysis, the major ones, which
accounted for 47% of the total extract, were identified as
actin, collagen and myosin. This was the first series of
extracts in which structural glycoprotein should have
appeared, and several bands in the gel remained unidentified,
which might perhaps have been structural glycoprotein.

The residue was further extracted four times with the
above buffer containing dithiothreitol, and this removed a
further 4% of the dry weight of the tissue. The picture on
PAGE was very similar to that of the guanidinium extract,
the only prominent bands being due to actin, collagen and
myosin.

Lastly the residue was extracted with 0.1M-NaOH but this
extract produced no discrete bands on PAGE.

However, since structural glycoprotein has more often
been prepared after initial removal of collagen, the authors
explored the three treatments of bacterial collagenase
digestion, autoclaving, and extraction with trichloracetic
acid. Each of these three steps was followed by extraction
of the residue with the guanidinium chloride-dithiothreitol
buffer. PAGE of extracts showed that both autoclaving and
trichloracetic acid treatment caused extensive degradation,
while removal of collagen with bacterial collagenase
resulted in an extract showing most of the bands present in
the corresponding extract from undigested aorta.

The authors conclude that no significant quantity of any
one unidentified protein was found which could have been
structural glycoprotein and which could account for reports
of large amounts of structural glycoprotein in aortas of
many species.

The argument here might be regarded at least partly as

a semantic one, since it is possible to define structural
glycoproteins in two different ways.   Firstly, they could
be defined as the non-collagenous, non-elastin, non-
proteoglycan fraction extractable from connective tissues by
chaotropic agents such as guanidinium chloride or urea,
usually after removal of collagen.   On the other hand, a
structural glycoprotein might be defined more precisely as
a distinct molecular species with specific properties.
There never has been a rigid decision by connective tissue
biochemists.   However, if we consider the first definition,
then Bach and Bentley (1980) are asserting that aorta
structural glycoprotein is largely actin.   On the basis of
the second definition, their findings mean that if aorta
structural glycoprotein exists, then it is only a minor
component.

A complementary method of unravelling the true
situation is undoubtedly a study of macromolecules actually
secreted by connective tissue cells.   In a preliminary
report Moczar et al (1979) described the secretion of
glycoproteins by rabbit aorta smooth muscle cells in culture.
Cells were incubated with ^{14}C-glucosamine, ^{3}H-fucose and
^{14}C-mannose for 18 hours followed by sequential treatment
with dithiothreitol - 0.2mM-CaCl$_2$ - 0.5mM-ATP pH 7.5,
5M-guanidinium chloride - 0.1% EDTA, bacterial collagenase
and finally guanidinium chloride-EDTA again.   Little
material was extracted by the first solvent, but the second
extracted four periodate-Schiff positive components of
mol. wts. 220 000, 170 000, 70 000 and 36 000.   All were
labelled with the three radioactive sugars.   Glycoproteins
released by bacterial collagenase had mol. wts. of 230 000,
150 000 and 36 000, and the 150 000 mol. wt. component
released a 70 000 fragment on PAGE.   The second
guanidinium extract contained glycoproteins of mol. wt.
220 000, 170 000 and 50 000.   It seems likely that the
220 000 mol. wt. component is fibronectin, the 170 000
mol. wt. glycoprotein is microfibrillar protein, while the
lowest mol. wt. constituent might be the carboxyl terminal
extension from procollagen.

In another study Jones et al (1979) demonstrated that
rat smooth muscle cells in culture secreted a fucosylated
glycoprotein having mol. wt. 250 000 and two other proteins
of mol. wts. 72 000 and 45 000.   The glycoprotein was
similar to fibronectin, while the other two proteins were
thought to be tropoelastin (72 000) and a collagenous peptide

similar to that known as CP45.

The macromolecules shown to be secreted in both these studies probably would have been classified previously as structural glycoproteins, but now as our knowledge advances we can be more precise about their origin and function.

CONCLUDING REMARKS

One of the most important questions we have to consider is whether there is, in most connective tissues, a protein or family of proteins, not fibronectin and not microfibriller protein, which may truly be described as structural glycoproteins. There is little evidence that this is so. The case for structural glycoproteins seems to be declining somewhat at a time when, with increasing studies on secretion of proteins by cells in culture, evidence for their existence should be accumulating.

It is now becoming apparent that intracellular proteins may be extracted from extracellular matrices under mild conditions. For example, a protein of mol. wt. about 60 000 isolated in this way might in fact be β subunit of prolyl hydroxylase. The extraction of intracellular proteins actin and myosin from aorta by Bach and Bentley (1980) may be explained in two ways. Firstly, these are truly intracellular proteins, but the initial homogenisation and extraction conditions result in the rupture of smooth muscle cells with release of intracellular contents (the presence of nucleic acid in guanidinium chloride extracts is not unknown). Secondly, perhaps actin and myosin are present extracellularly in smooth muscle. Chen et al (1978) identified actin in matrix prepared from chick fibroblasts. The extracellular presence of prolyl and lysyl hydroxylases and galactosyl and glucosyl transferases has already been discussed (Anderson, 1980). However, these enzymes are already halfway there in the sense that they are located on the internal face of the cisternae of the endoplasmic reticulum.

Aalto M, Potila M, Kulonen E (1979). Glycoproteins from experimental granulation tissue and their effects on collagen synthesis in embryonic chick cells. Biochim Biophys Acta 587:606-617.

Anderson JC (1976). Glycoproteins of the connective tissue matrix. In Hall DA, Jackson DS (eds): "International Review of Connective Tissue Research" New York: Academic Press, Vol 7:251-322.

Anderson JC (1980). Recent advances in the study of connective tissue glycoproteins. In Robert A, Robert L (eds): "Biochimie des Tissus Conjonctifs Normaux et Pathologiques": Editions CNRS, tome II, p 195-199.

Bach PR, Bentley JP (1980). Structural glycoprotein, fact or artefact. Connect Tiss Res 7:185-196

Berg RA, Kedersha NL, Guzman NA (1979). Purification and partial characterisation of the two nonidentical subunits of prolyl hydroxylase. J Biol Chem 254:3111-3118.

Bowness JM (1978). Association of structural glycoproteins with lipids or lipoprotein. Atherosclerosis 31:403-408.

Chen LB, Murray A, Segal RA, Bushnell A, Walsh ML (1978). Studies on intercellular LETS glycoprotein matrices. Cell 14:377-391.

Chichester CO, Fuller GC, Mo Cha CJ (1979). Turnover of prolyl hydroxylase and an immunologically related protein in rabbit tissue. Biochim Biophys Acta 586:341-356.

Davidson JM, McEneany LSG, Bornstein P (1979). Procollagen processing: limited proteolysis of carboxyl terminal extension peptides by a cathepsin-like protease secreted by tendon fibroblasts. Eur J Biochem 100:551-558.

Jones PA, Scott-Burden T, Gevers W (1979). Glycoprotein, elastin and collagen secretion by rat smooth muscle cells. Proc Natl Acad Sci 76:353-357.

Kagan HM, Sullivan KA, Olsson TO, Cronlund AL (1979). Purification and properties of four species of lysyl oxidase from bovine aorta. Biochem J 177:203-214.

Kao WW-Y, Chou K-LL (1980). CRP, immunologically cross-reacting protein of prolyl hydroxylase. Its role in assembly of active prolyl hydroxylase and cellular localisation in L-929 fibroblasts. Arch Biochem Biophys 199:147-157.

Kaplan A, Fischer D, Achord D, Sly W (1977). Phosphohexosyl recognition is a general characteristic of pinocytosis of lysosomal glycosidases by human fibroblasts. J Clin Invest 60:1088-1093.

Mbuyi JM, Dequeker J, Leuven KU (1980). A comparison of the organic matrix from rat bone and rat skin. Poster: this meeting.

Miller RL, Varner HH (1979). Purification and enzymatic properties of lysyl hydroxylase from fetal porcine skin. Biochemistry 18:5928-5932.

Moczar M, Moczar E, Robert L (1977).   Structural
  glycoprotein from the media of pig aorta.   Aggregation
  of S-carboxamidomethyl subunits.   Biochimie 59:141-151.
Moczar M, Phan-Dinh-Tuy B, Moczar E (1979).   Glycoproteins
  associated to the collagen-elastin matrix of aorta.
  In Schauer R, Boer P, Buddecke E, Kramer MF,
  Vliegenthart JFG, Wiegandt (eds): "Glycoconjugates:
  Proceedings of the Fifth International Symposium"
  Stuttgart: Georg Thieme, p 557-558.
Randoux A, Maquart F, Cornillet-Stoupy J, Szymanowicz G,
  Borel JP (1978).   Influence of structural glycoproteins
  on the biosynthesis of collagen by fibroblasts in culture.
  In Robert A, Robert L (eds): "Biochimie des Tissus
  Conjonctifs Normaux et Pathologiques" Paris: Editions
  CNRS, tome I, p 257-8.
Serafini-Fracassini A, Ventrella G, Griffiths R, Hinnie J
  (1980).   Characterisation of a self associating
  glycoprotein from bovine ligamentum nuchae exhibiting dual
  amine oxidase activity.   Poster: this meeting.
Shipp DW, Bowness JM (1975).   Insoluble non-collagenous
  cartilage glycoproteins with aggregating subunits.
  Biochim Biophys Acta 379:282-294.
Swann DA, Sotman S, Dixon M, Brooks C (1977).   The
  isolation and partial characterisation of the major
  glycoprotein from the articular lubricating fraction from
  bovine synovial fluid.   Biochem J 161:473-485.
Swann DA, Mintz G (1979).   The isolation and properties of
  a second glycoprotein (LGP-II) from the articular
  lubricating fraction from bovine synovial fluid.
  Biochem J 179:465-471.
Tuderman L, Kivirikko KI, Prockop DJ (1978).   Partial
  purification and characterisation of a neutral protease
  which cleaves the N-terminal propeptides from procollagen.
  Biochemistry 17:2948-2954.

Connective Tissue Research:
Chemistry, Biology, and Physiology, Pages 73–86
© 1981 Alan R. Liss, Inc., 150 Fifth Avenue, New York, N.Y. 10011

STRUCTURAL GLYCOPROTEINS OF CONNECTIVE TISSUE

Jacqueline Labat-Robert

Laboratoire de Biochimie du Tissu Conjonctif
(GR CNRS No 40) Faculté de Médecine,
8 rue du Général Sarrail
94010 Créteil-Cedex, France

I - GENERALITIES

Connective tissues contain glycoconjugates different
from collagens and proteoglycans. These are now generally
designated as structural glycoproteins (SGP)(A.M. Robert et
al., 1970).

These macromolecules are synthesized in situ by fibroblasts or other differentiated mesenchymal cells (such as
chondrocytes, smooth muscle cells of vascular walls)(Robert
and Parlebas, 1965 ; Kern et al., 1976 ; Moczar et al., 1976;
Robert et al., 1973), thus differing from plasma glycoproteins which are mostly synthesized in the liver. It should
be observed nevertheless that some structural glycoproteins
may be present in biological fluids (plasma, cerebrospinal
fluid, amniotic fluid) as for example cold insoluble globulin (CIG)(Morrison et al., 1948 ; Mosesson et al., 1970),
antigelatin factor (Dessau et al., 1978a).

SGP-s are very ancient molecules. They appear during
phylogenesis at the same time as collagen, that is from the
first metazoans : the Porifera. Five years ago, in our laboratory, low molecular weight SGP-s have been isolated and
characterized for the first time from horny sponges (Junqua
et al., 1975a, b ; Junqua, 1979). The overall composition
of these glycoproteins appeared to be very close to that of
the SGP-s isolated from vertebrate sources. More recently,
using a high titer antihuman cold insoluble globulin antiserum and immunofluorescence staining, we could also demonstrate the presence of a fibronectin-like protein in fresh

water sponge cells (Ephydatia mulleri)(Labat-Robert et al.,
1979). A strong immune fluorescence was observed on the
membranes of epithelial cells, all over flagellate cells
(choanocytes) which ensure the circulation of water through
the animal and fibroblast-like cells (lophocytes) which
synthesize collagen.

Thus, structural glycoproteins appear during the phylogenesis before proteoglycans which are present only in
higher invertebrates, and before elastin which has been
found until now, only in vertebrates.

II - METHODS OF ISOLATION

As underlined by Anderson in his review (Anderson, 1976)
there are four major problems in the isolation of structural
glycoproteins : their release and separation from the
collagen-matrix, their separation from proteoglycans, their
separation from serum proteins and cells, and lastly the
danger of possible degradation by proteases and glycosidases.

An example of the preparation of SGP-s is given in
Figure 1.

Tissue

1) Wash in NaCl 0.9 % to eliminate serum proteins

2) Delipidation in alternate extractions in
   acetone and n-butanol (important for aorta,
   not necessary for cornea)

3) $MgCl_2$ 2M,
   3 x extractions of 24 h at 4°C

4) Guanidine HCl 5M
   3 x extractions of 24 h at 4°C

5) Collagenase CLSPA Worthington, exempt of
   non specific proteases
   24h at 22°C under toluene wash with buffer

6) Guanidine HCl 5M
   2-mercaptoethanol 0.1M (or dithiothreitol 0.05M)
   3 x 24h at 4°C, wash in H_2O

7) Final residue : elastin (fibrous, polymeric)

Figure 1

Most authors use purified bacterial collagenase for the "solubilisation" of the insoluble polymeric stroma. Dispersion for the separation from collagens of the polymeric stroma in detergents, metal complexing agents (EDTA) or concentrated salt solutions is also used (Anderson, 1976 ; Moczar and Moczar, 1981). Equilibrium density centrifugation in cesium chloride can be used for the separation from proteoglycans, extraction by physiological saline for the removal of serum proteins, with the necessary presence of protease inhibitors in the extraction buffers.

III - PHYSICOCHEMICAL PROPERTIES

The structural glycoprotein family is a very heterogenous one as it can be judged from the dispersion of the molecular weights reported which vary from 16,000 for SGP-s isolated from rabbit skin (Randoux et al., 1976) to 850,000 for laminin (Rohde et al., 1979).

The amino acid composition of structural glycoproteins shows a high content in dicarboxylic amino acid, the presence of cystein and a relatively high proportion of aliphatic amino acids (Table 1). Nevertheless this composition is similar to that of several glycoproteins of other origin.

The carbohydrate content varies largely from hardly detectable quantities in a SGP isolated from rabbit skin by Stoupy et al. (1972) to 15 % in laminin (Timpl et al., 1979b). The carbohydrate residues are N-acetylglucosamine, galactose, mannose, fucose and sialic acid. Sometimes N-acetylgalactosamine and glucose have been reported. They are essentially N-glycosylglycoproteins. As far as it can be judged from the presently available information they do not differ from plasma N-glycosylglycoproteins. Structural glycoproteins may exist intracellularly and at or near the cell membrane in connective tissues. They are present free or associated to other components in the intercellular matrix. Some may be linked to fibrous proteins such as collagens (fibronectin) or elastin (microfibrillar glyco-proteins), others are linked to proteoglycans (link-glyco-proteins).

For all these reasons, the concept was formulated in our laboratory of a possible role of structural glycoproteins in the morphogenesis of connective tissue, in the positioning the cells in the intercellular matrix (Robert and Robert, 1974). As finally the structure and function

TABLE 1

Amino acid composition of several connective tissue structural glycoprotein preparations. All values expressed as residues per 1,000 residues.

	Calf cornea	Pig aorta	Spongia Officinalis	Metridium dianthus sea anemone	Rabbit dermis	
	Robert and Comte (1968)	Moczar and Robert (1970)	Junqua et al.(1975)	Katzman (1972)	Timpl et al.(1968)	Stoupy et al.(1972)
ASP	102	90	98	109	96.7	94
THR	51	54	60	56	59.6	59
SER	59	57	47	56	60.8	54
GLU	113	100	101	124	131.3	161
PRO	57	52	52	51	60.0	45
GLY	105	88	90	73	63.9	71
ALA	70	81	87	75	73.8	91
1/2 CYST	15	27	9	21	7.1	–
VAL	86	74	76	64	58.8	59
MET	11	1	27	22	21.6	26
ILE	47	43	64	47	58.0	66
LEU	47	77	83	78	91.9	101
TYR	17	28	32	32	27.9	34
PHE	38	31	46	35	39.3	41
TRP	*	ND	**	ND	ND	16
LYS	44	57	48	74	70.5	42
HIS	15	22	20	17	21.1	10
ARG	60	46	60	58	57.3	29

* 2 % of total protein.   ** 0.8 % of total protein.

TABLE 1 (CONTINUED)

Amino acid composition of several connective tissue structural glycoprotein preparations. All values expressed as residues per 1,000 residues

	Puppy cartilage Shipp and Bowness (1975)	Bovine Achilles tendon Anderson and Jackson (1972)	Human fibronectin Yamada et al. (1978)	Laminin Timpl et al. (1979)
ASP	123	107	92	109
THR	52	65	97	58
SER	56	63	68	77
GLU	116	122	116	122
PRO	63	67	76	53
GLY	98	57	80	93
ALA	67	75	43	76
1/2 CYST	25	41	26	30
VAL	68	72	81	48
MET	10	9	11	14
ILE	44	33	44	42
LEU	94	83	57	92
TYR	26	32	45	27
PHE	36	38	27	31
TRP	ND	ND	28	ND
LYS	50	71	36	52
HIS	21	21	21	24
ARG	54	44	52	50

of multicellular organisms depend on the stabilised three-dimensional topological arrangement of individual cells to form tissues and of tissues to form organs, one can under-stand henceforth the great importance of intercellular matrix in general and of structural glycoproteins in particular as the main integrators of cells in the organism.

We can examplify this important role of SGP-s bv the example of fibronectin.

IV - FIBRONECTIN

This term : Fibronectin, designates a group of glyco-proteins composed of subunits of about 220,000 daltons, sharing some biological properties and exhibiting common immunological characteristics. Some of these glycoproteins are listed in Table 2.

1. Cold insoluble globulin
2. Antigelatin factor
3. Microfibrillar glycoprotein
4. α_2 SB opsonic glycoprotein
5. Galactoprotein a
6. Surface fibroblast antigen
7. L.E.T.S.
8. Cell surface protein
9. L1 band
10. Zeta protein
11. Band 1 protein
12. Collagen dependent cell attachment protein
13. Cell spreading factor
14. Major fibroblast glycoprotein
15. Cell adhesion factor

Table 2 - Fibronectins

Some of these fibronectins are soluble (cold insoluble globulin, antigelatin factor, for example) and are present in blood plasma and other biological fluids. Others are insoluble and are present in the intercellular matrix. The cells that express this surface protein lie close to sup-portive structures and extrude it into the intercellular matrix as fibers (Hedman et al., 1978). Fibronectin is extensively distributed in tissues : it is associated with basement membranes, including embryonic skin, trophoblast and alveolar basement membranes (Bray, 1978), spleen, intestines, liver, thyroid gland and the sarcolemma of striated muscle (Stenman and Vaheri, 1978). In vitro, many cell types are able to produce fibronectin : fibroblastic cells, astroglial cells, endothelial cells, some epithelial cells, macrophages (Vaheri et al., 1980).

In cell culture, fibronectin is synthesized as a monomeric polypeptide chain. As soon as it can be detected in the cell it contains carbohydrate chains. Rapidly the monomeric chain dimerizes inside the cell, and appears as a dimer on the cell surface and in the culture medium (Choi and Hynes, 1979). There is a continuous shedding of fibronectin from the cell to the medium by a mechanism which is not yet understood.

Fibronectin is a high molecular weight (450,000) glycoprotein, formed by two subunits covalently linked by disulphide bridges. The molecular weights of the two subunits are thought to be equal, but no conclusive evidence is yet available to support this proposition. It contains 4 to 5 % of carbohydrates. Some authors have studied the glycan structure (Takasaki et al., 1979 ; Wrann, 1978 ; Carter and Hakomori, 1979). There is a microheterogeneity in the carbohydrate chains.Nevertheless the glycan chains have the same general structure as other N-glycosyl plasma glycoproteins; they appear to belong to the L-type defined by Strecker and Montreuil (1979) i.e. to the N-acetyllactosamine type with the _invariant_ non specific carbohydrate core formed by the β-glycosidic bond of a mannotriose to a di-N-acetylchitobiose residue, linked itself to an asparagyl residue. This core is substituted by a variable number of N-acetyllactosaminyl residues, sialic acid and/or fucose residues.

Fibronectin presents some interesting properties such as specific and strong interactions with collagens, fibrin, fibrinogen and proteoglycans.

The interaction with collagen has been extensively studied (Jilek and Hormann, 1978 ; Gold et al., 1979 ; Furie et al., 1980 ; Furie and Rifkin, 1980 ; Balian et al., 1980; Kleinman et al., 1979a and b ; Dessau et al., 1978b ; Hahn and Yamada, 1978). Its specificity appears to be due to the existence of a well defined collagen binding site on fibronectin and of a well defined fibronectin binding site present on all the collagen types studied. A cell binding site was demonstrated on fibronectin which is different from the collagen binding site (Ruoslahti and Hayman, 1979).

Some other binding regions appear to exist also on fibronectin, namely for proteoglycans and/or glycosamino-glycans (Ruoslahti et al., 1979 ; Culp et al., 1979). These observations suggest the importance of fibronectin in vivo. Furthermore in connective tissues, it appears that fibronectin and collagen frequently codistribute. Fibronectin may thus have an organizing role in cell-matrix interaction and in the organisation of the intercellular matrix.

The contention that fibronectin is important in directing cell to cell and cell-matrix interactions is supported also by the following experiments.

In culture, most malignant cells loose their surface fibronectin (Hynes et al., 1979). The reason of this loss is not yet completely understood. It could result from a decrease in the biosynthesis of fibronectin (Olden and Yamada, 1977), but this is not always the case (Parry et al., 1979), from an increase in protease levels (Yamada and Pouyssegur, 1978), or from a modification of the membrane receptors (Kleinman et al., 1979a). Whatever the cause may be, the result of the loss of surface fibronectin is a change in the cell morphology and in their adhesion properties. In vitro addition of purified fibronectin to transformed cells appears to restore their aberrant cell to cell and cell to matrix relationships, toward a normal behaviour (Olden and Yamada, 1977 ; Vaheri and Ruoslahti, 1975).

Another example of this role in cell to cell interaction was obtained during our study on the presence of a fibronectin-like protein in fresh water sponge cells (Labat-Robert et al., 1979). We wanted to know whether this protein could play a role in the reaggregation of dissociated sponge cells. After mechanical dissociation of cells, they reaggregate easily in a suspension medium containing Ca^{++} and Mg^{++}. We could inhibit this process by adding a highly diluted gelatin solution to the medium. Gelatin interacts with fibronectin on the cell surface and interferes with the cell to cell recognition process. We could also inhibit the reaggregation of the dissociated sponge cells by adding to the medium a highly diluted anti-human cold insoluble globulin antiserum. In this case, the inhibition decreased with the increasing dilution of the antiserum.

The behaviour of fibronectin has been studied towards the neutral proteases released from inflammatory cells, such as polymorphonuclear leukocytes. McDonald et al. (1979) could show that in vitro fibronectin is a sensitive target for these proteases. These results also suggest that the morphological and functional changes observed in the inflammatory processes may reflect fibronectin destruction, in addition to damage to other components of the intercellular matrix.

V - FIBRONECTIN IN SOLID HUMAN TUMORS

We started recently a systematic study of the distribution of fibronectin in solid human tumors (Labat-Robert et al., 1980a, b). One of the most generally recognized characteristics of solid human tumors is the profound modification of the normal tissue structure. Structure and function of normal tissues depend on the stable topological arrangement of individual cells into tissues, which is mediated by cell to cell and cell to matrix interactions and which is also the result of the "program" of synthesis of the macromolecules of the intercellular matrix (Robert and Robert, 1973).

Our data obtained with breast cancers, and other human tumors : bronchi, endometrium-prostatic tissue for example, confirm the existence of a strongly modified distribution pattern of fibronectin in human neoplastic tissues. Two kinds of tumors have been studied : carcinomas and sarcomas. In carcinomas, the loss of fibronectin, normally present on cell membranes and in basement membranes, is well correlated with the infiltration of the stroma by the malignant cells. In non-infiltrating carcinomas fibronectin is still detectable in the basal lamina, often as irregular strips. The disappearance of fibronectin corresponded to a progressive infiltrative process.

In sarcomas, fibronectin normally present on the cell surface of fibroblasts, muscle cells and adipocytes appears to be lost. By contrast in benign proliferations, fibronectin could be clearly visualized around the same cells. The persistence of the pericellular fibronectin appears to be a reliable marker of the benign proliferation particularly in pseudo-tumoral or inflammatory lesions of the soft tissues (Labat-Robert et al., 1980a).

From the above facts, it appears that structural glycoproteins play a key role in the morphogenesis and function of connective tissues. Over the last years, a real progress has been accomplished in our understanding of such processes, largely through the studies on fibronectin. The recent isolation of laminin (Timpl et al., 1979a, b ; Rohde et al.,

1979) and of several other SGP-s (Robert et al., 1976 ; Moczar and Moczar 1978 ; Junqua et al., 1979 ; Lafuma et al., 1979 ; Anderson, 1980 ; Robert, 1980) will significantly contribute to our knowledge of the important functions of intercellular matrix in normal and pathological conditions.

REFERENCES

Anderson JC (1976). Glycoproteins of the connective tissue matrix. Int Rev Connect Tissue Res 7:251.
Anderson JC (1980). Recent advances in the study of connective tissue glycoproteins. In Robert AM, Robert L (eds) "Biochimie des Tissus Conjonctifs Normaux et Pathologiques" Colloques Internationaux du CNRS N° 287, Paris: CNRS, p. 195.
Anderson JC, Jackson DS (1972). The isolation of glycoproteins from bovine Achilles tendon and their interaction with collagen. Biochem J 127:179.
Balian G, Glick EM, Bornstein P (1980). Location of a collagen-binding domain in fibronectin. J Biol Chem 255:3234
Bray BA (1978). Presence of fibronectin in basement membranes and acidic structural glycoproteins from human placenta and lung. Ann NY Acad Sci 312:142.
Carter WG, Hakomori SI (1979). Isolation of galactoprotein a from hamster embryo fibroblasts and characterization of the carbohydrate unit. Biochemistry 18:730.
Choi MG, Hynes RO (1979). Biosynthesis and processing of fibronectin in NIL 8 Hamster cells. J Biol Chem 254:12050.
Culp LA, Murray BA, Rollins BJ (1979). Fibronectin and proteoglycans as determinants of cell-substratum adhesion. J Supramol Structure 11:401.
Dessau W, Jilek F, Adelmann BC, Hörmann H (1978a). Similarity of antigelatin factor and cold-insoluble globulin. Biochim Biophys Acta 533:227.
Dessau W, Adelmann BC, Timpl R, Martin GR (1978b). Identification of the sites in collagen α-chains that bind serum-antigelatin factor (cold-insoluble globulin). Biochem J 169:55.
Furie MB, Frey AB, Rifkin DB (1980). Location of a gelatin-binding region of human plasma fibronectin. J Biol Chem 255:4391.
Furie MB, Rifkin DB (1980). Proteolytically derived fragments of human plasma fibronectin and their localization within the intact molecule. J Biol Chem 255:3134
Gold LI, Garcia-Pardo A, Frangione B, Franklin EC, Pearlstein E (1979). Subtilisin and cyanogen bromide cleavage products of fibronectin that retain gelatin-binding activity. Proc

Ntl Acad Sci (USA) 76:4803.

Grinnell F, Feld M, Minter D (1980). Fibroblast adhesion to fibrinogen and fibrin substrata-requirement for cold insoluble globulin (plasma fibronectin). Cell 19:517.

Hahn LHE, Yamada KM (1978). Isolation and biological characterization of active fragments of the adhesive glycoprotein fibronectin. Cell 18:1043.

Hedman K, Vaheri A, Wartiovaara J (1978). External fibronectin of cultured human fibroblasts is predominantly a matrix protein. J Cell Biol 76:748.

Hynes RO, Destree AT, Perkins ME, WagnerDD (1979) Cell surface proteins and oncogenic transformation. J Supramol Struct 11:95.

Jilek F, Hörmann H (1978). Cold insoluble globulin (fibronectin), IV. Affinity to soluble collagen of various types. Hoppe-Seyler's Z Physiol Chem 359:247.

Junqua S, Fayolle J, Robert L (1975a).Isolation and characterization of structural glycoproteins from sponges. In Peeters H (ed) : "Protides of the Biological Fluids," Pergamon Press, Oxford/New York 22:337.

Junqua S, Fayolle J, Robert L (1975b). Structural glycoproteins from sponge intercellular matrix. Comp Biochem Physiol 50B:305.

Junqua S, Robert L (1979). Fractionation of sponge structural-glycoproteins by affinity chromatography on lectins. In Gregory J, Jeanloz R (eds) "Glycoconjugate Research," Academic Press 1:177.

Katzman RL (1972). Structural glycoprotein from Metridium dianthus connective tissue. Life Sci 11:131.

Kern P, Regnault F, Robert L (1976). Biochemical and ultrastructural study of human diabetic conjunctiva. Biomedecine 24:32.

Kleinman HK, Martin GR, Fishman PH (1979a). Ganglioside inhibition of fibronectin-mediated cell adhesion to collagen. Proc Natl Acad Sci USA 76:3367.

Kleinman HK, Hewitt AT, Murray JC, Liotta LA, Rennard SI, Pennypacker JP, McGoodwin EB, Martin GR, Fishman PH (1979b). Cellular and metabolic specificity in the interaction of adhesion proteins with collagen and with cells. J Supramol Struct 11:69.

Labat-Robert J, Pavans de Ceccatty M, Robert L, Auger C, Lethias C, Garonne R (1979). Surface glycoproteins of sponge cells : presence of a fibronectin-like protein on differentiated sponge cell membranes, its role in cell aggregation. In Schauer R, Boer P, Buddecke E, Kramer MF, Vliegenthart JFG, Wiegandt H (eds) "Glycoconjugates," Georg Thieme Pub Stuttgart, p. 431

Labat-Robert J, Birembaut P, Adnet JJ, Mercantini F, Robert

L (1980a). Loss of fibronectin in human breast cancer. Cell Biol Interntl Rep 4:609.

Labat-Robert J, Birembaut P, Robert L, Adnet JJ (1980b). Modification of fibronectin distribution pattern in solid human tumors. Invest Cell Pathol, in print.

Lafuma C, Moczar M, Robert L (1979). Protéines non collagé-niques de la matrice intersticielle pulmonaire du rat. Bull Europ Physiopathol Respiratoire 15:38.

MacDonald JA, Baum BJ, Rosenberg DM, Kelman JA, Brin SC, Crystal RG (1979). Destruction of a major extracellular adhesive glycoprotein (fibronectin) of human fibroblasts by neutral proteases from polymorphonuclear leukocyte granules. Lab Invest 40:350.

Moczar M, Robert L (1970). Extraction and fractionation of the media of aorta. Atherosclerosis 11:7.

Moczar M, Allard R, Ouzilou J, Robert L, Bouissou H, Julian M, Pieraggi MT (1976). Structural and biochemical altera-tions of human diabetic dermis studied by 3H-lysine incorporation and microscopy. Path Biol 24:329.

Moczar M, Moczar E (1978). Glycoproteins from the aorta. Path Biol 26:64.

Moczar E, Moczar M (1981). Methodology of connective tissue research. In Robert L (ed). "Frontiers of Matrix Biology," Vol. 10, Karger, Basel, in print.

Morrison PR, Edsall JT, Miller SG (1948). Preparation and properties of serum and plasma proteins. XVIII The sepa-ration of purified fibrinogen from fraction 1 of human plasma. J Am Chem Soc 70:3103.

Mosesson MW, Umfleet RA (1970). The cold-insoluble globulin of human plasma. I. Purification primary characterization, and relationship to fibrinogen and other cold-insoluble fraction components. J Biol Chem 245:5728.

Olden K, Yamada KM (1977). Mechanism of the decrease of the major cell surface protein of chick embryo fibroblasts after transformation. Cell 11:957.

Parry G, Soo WJ, Bissell MJ (1979). The uncoupled regula-tion of fibronectin and collagen synthesis in Rous sar-coma virus transformed avian tendon cells. J Biol Chem 254:11763.

Randoux A, Cornillet-Stoupy J, Desanti M, Borel JP (1976). Isolement et caractérisation de deux subunités constitu-tives de glycoprotéines de structure du tissu sous-cutané de lapin. Biochim Biophys Acta 446:77.

Robert L, Parlebas J (1963). Biosynthèse in vitro des glyco-protéines de la cornée. Bull Soc Chim Biol 47:1853.

Robert L, Comte P (1968). Amino acid composition of struc-tural glycoproteins. Life Sci 7:493.

Robert AM, Robert B, Robert L (1970). Chemical and physical

properties of structural glycoproteins. In Balazs EA (ed) "Chemistry and Molecular Biology of the Intercellular Matrix," Vol. 1, Academic Press London, p. 237.

Robert L, Junqua S, Robert AM, Moczar M, Robert B (1973). In vitro incorporation of labelled precursors in the macromolecules of the polymeric stroma of normal and pathological arterial wall. In Kulonen K, Pikkarainen J (eds) "Biology of Fibroblast," New York: Academic Press, p. 637.

Robert B, Robert L (1973). Aging of connective tissues. General considerations. In Robert L (ed) "Frontiers of Matrix Biology," Vol. 1, Basel: Karger, p. 1.

Robert L, Robert B (1974). Structural glycoproteins of connective tissue : their role in morphogenesis and immunopathology. In Fricke R, Hartmann F (eds): "Connective Tissues Biochemistry and Pathology," Berlin: Springer Verlag, p. 240.

Robert L, Junqua S, Moczar M (1976). Structural glycoproteins of the intercellular matrix. In Robert AM, Robert L (eds): "Frontiers of Matrix Biology," Basel, Karger, Vol. 3, p. 113.

Robert L (1980). Structural glycoproteins : the fourth family of matrix macromolecules. In Robert AM, Robert L (eds): Colloque Internationaux du CNRS N° 287 "Biochimie des Tissus Conjonctifs Normaux et Pathologiques" Paris: CNRS, p. 189.

Rohde H, Wick G, Timpl R (1979). Immunochemical characterization of the basement membrane glycoprotein laminin. Eur J Biochem 102:195.

Ruoslahti E, Hayman EG (1979). Two active sites with different characteristics in fibronectin. Febs Lett 97:221.

Ruoslahti E, Pekkala A, Engvall E (1979). Effect of dextran sulfate on fibronectin-collagen interaction. Febs Lett 107:51.

Shipp DW, Bowness M (1975). Insoluble non-collagenous cartilage glycoproteins with aggregating subunits. Biochim Biophys Acta 379:282.

Stathakis NE, Mosesson MW (1977). Interactions among heparin, cold-insoluble globulin and fibrinogen in formation of the heparin-precipitable fraction of plasma. J Clin Invest 60:855.

Stenman S, Vaheri A (1978). Distribution of a major connective tissue protein, fibronectin, in normal human tissues. J Exp Med 147:1054.

Stoupy J, Vieillard A, Desanti M, Borel JP, Randoux A (1972). Composition de certaines fractions de glycoproteines de structure de l'hypoderme de lapin. CR Acad Sci Paris 275:2997.

Strecker G, Montreuil J (1979). Glycoprotéines et glycoprotéinoses. Biochimie 61:1199.

Takasaki S, Yamashita K, Suzuki K, Iwanaga S, Kobata A (1979). The sugar chains of cold-insoluble globulin, a protein related to fibronectin. J Biol Chem 254:8548.

Timpl R, Wolff I, Weiser M (1968). A new class of structural proteins from connective tissue. Biochim Biophys Acta 168:168.

Timpl R, Rohde H, Gehron-Robey P, Rennard SI, Foidart JM, Martin GR (1979a). Laminin - a glycoprotein from basement membranes. J Biol Chem 254:9933.

Timpl R, Rohde H, Ott-Ullbricht U, Risteli L, Bächeriger HP (1979b). Chemical characterization of laminin,a major glycoprotein of basement membrane. In Schauer R, Boer P, Buddecke E, Kramer MF, Vliegenthart JFG, Wiegandt H (eds): "Glycoconjugates," Stuttgart: G. Thieme, p. 145.

Vaheri A, Alitalo K, Hedman K, Kurkinen M, Saksela O, Vartio T (1980). Fibronectin and its loss in malignant transformation. In Robert AM, Robert L (eds): Colloques Internationaux du CNRS N° 287 "Biochimie des Tissus Conjonctifs Normaux et Pathologiques," Paris: CNRS, p. 249.

Vaheri A, Ruoslahti E (1975). Fibroblast surface antigen produced but not retained by virus-transformed human cells. J Exp Med 142:530.

Wrann M (1978). Methylation analysis of the carbohydrate portion of fibronectin isolated from human plasma. Biochem Biophys Res Comm 84:269.

Yamada KM, Olden K, Pastan I (1978). Transformation-sensitive cell surface protein : isolation, characterization and role in cellular morphology and adhesion. Ann NY Acad Sci 312:256.

Yamada KM, Pouyssegur J (1978). Cell surface glycoproteins and malignant transformation. Biochimie 60:1221.

Connective Tissue Research:
Chemistry, Biology, and Physiology, Pages 87-112
© 1981 Alan R. Liss, Inc., 150 Fifth Avenue, New York, N.Y. 10011

RECENT ADVANCES IN THE BIOCHEMISTRY OF HYALURONIC ACID IN CARTILAGE

R.M. Mason

Dept. Biochemistry, Charing Cross Hospital
Medical School, University of London,
London, W6 8RF, U.K.

Hyaluronic acid*, a linear chain glycosaminoglycan having a repeating unit structure $[(1{\to}4)-\beta-D-glucuronosyl-(1{\to}3)-\beta-D-N-acetyglucosaminyl]_n$, is widely distributed in connective tissues. The molecular weight of the chain is variable but can exceed 1×10^6.

Recent investigations have shown that HA is an important component of cartilages in which it may have both structural and regulatory functions. This review attempts to outline what is presently known about the molecule in cartilage and summarises our recent attempts to study its biosynthesis by chondrocytes in primary cell cultures.

HYALURONIC ACID CONTENT OF CARTILAGE

Seno & Anno (1960) were the first to show that HA was present in whale hyaline cartilage. The introduction of specific microfractionation methods for glycosaminoglycans, based on the solubility of their cetyl pyridinium salts (Scott, 1960) subsequently led to the discovery that HA was present in many types of cartilage.

Antonopoulos et $al.$ (1964) applied the method to the analysis of nasal septum cartilage from young (<3 yr) and old (>8 yr) horses and reported that HA-glucosamine constituted just over 0.4% of the dry tissue weight (equivalent to 0.7-

*Abbreviation. HA, Hyaluronic acid, normally present in tissues as sodium hyaluronate.

0.8% HA). The dry tissue content of chondroitin sulphate and keratan sulphate decreased and increased respectively with age, but HA levels remained virtually unchanged in the two groups. In a study where serial sections of horse nasal septum were analysed, the HA-fraction was uniformly distributed throughout the tissue (Szirmai, 1967).

A similar fractionation of dog epiphyseal plate cartilage showed that it too contained small amounts of HA (∼0.6-1.3% HA of organic dry weight) (Hjertquist, 1964a). The HA content of rachitic epiphyseal cartilage was reported as higher than in normal dogs. In contrast to nasal cartilage, microchemical analysis of different zones of epiphyseal plates suggested that the HA was not uniformly distributed through the tissue (Hjertquist, 1964b). In normal plates, the concentration was highest in the zone of provisional calcification whilst in rachitic and healing cartilage it was highest in the hypertrophic zone. Larsson *et al.* (1973) investigated the glycosaminoglycans of calf epiphyseal cartilage and also reported increasing concentrations of HA toward the calcification front, relative to chondroitin sulphate.

Other hyaline cartilages in which the HA content has been quantitated include pig laryngeal (0.35 mg/g wet wt, equivalent to about 1.2 mg/g dry wt) pig nasal (1.0-1.2 mg/g dry wt), bovine nasal (0.9-1.3 mg/g dry wt) and bovine articular cartilage (∼2.0-4.7 mg/g dry wt) (Hardingham & Muir, 1974; Pearson & Mason, 1979; Thonar *et al.*, 1978). Several human cartilages have also been investigated, particularly with respect to age-related changes in HA content (see below).

Fibrous and elastic cartilages also contain HA. Solheim (1965) found small amounts in the fibrocartilage of adult human meniscus, an observation later confirmed by McNicol & Roughley (1980). Solheim (1968) reported that equal amounts of HA and chondroitin sulphate were present in the elastic cartilage of human epiglottis. In pig epiglottal cartilage, HA contributes only 1.3% of the total uronic acid and accounts for 0.9 mg/g dry tissue weight. However, the ratio of HA:chondroitin sulphate is higher than in pig nasal or bovine nasal cartilage (HA = 0.4% total uronic acid) because the epiglottal cartilage has a relatively low chondroitin sulphate content (Pearson & Mason, 1979). Rabbit ear cartilage, another elastic tissue, is also relatively enriched in HA (Wusteman & Gillard, 1977).

EFFECT OF AGE ON CARTILAGE HA CONTENT

Several studies have suggested that the HA content of hyaline cartilage increases with age. Bayliss & Ali (1978) provided indirect evidence for this in human articular cartilage. In human costal cartilage, HA increased from 1.0-1.2 mg/g dry wt in infancy to over 2.0 mg/g in the fifth decade and later (Pearson & Mason, 1979). Thonar *et al.* (1978) investigated the HA content of bovine articular cartilage at different ages. The concentration rose from ∿0.06 μmoles glucosamine (HA)/100 mg wet tissue in the foetus to a maximum of 0.39 μmoles/100 mg in 3-10 year old steers. The water content of the tissue dropped from ∿90% to ∿70% during this time. There was little change in the cartilage HA concentration during foetal development.

The intervertebral disc is widely regarded as a specialised cartilagenous tissue. Hardingham & Adams (1976) used a proteoglycan-binding assay to measure the HA concentration of human lumbar disc which rose from 0.055% of the wet wt of the nucleus pulposus at 5 years to 0.273% in a 65-year-old specimen. The concentration in the annulus fibrosis increased less dramatically with age. Local changes in HA concentration across the disc paralleled changes in proteoglycan concentration.

Assessing the significance of changes in the HA concentration in ageing cartilage is complicated by simultaneous changes occurring in other matrix macromolecules. The proteoglycans become smaller as a result of a decrease in the size of the chondroitin sulphate attachment region (Inerot *et al.*, 1978). The keratan sulphate-rich region and the HA-binding region of the core protein remain comparatively constant and for this reason Inerot *et al.* proposed that the keratan sulphate content of cartilage is a better indicator of the molar concentration of proteoglycans in the tissue than chondroitin sulphate. However, Sweet *et al.* (1979) have shown that there is an increased substitution of keratan sulphate chains on to the small proteoglycans of old tissue. Thus, with the added complication of heterogeneity (Pearson & Mason, 1978), it is difficult to calculate the exact molar concentration of proteoglcans in the tissue at any given age. Nevertheless, it seems likely that there is an increase in the number of proteoglycans in the tissue with age and it is possible that the increases in HA concentration parallel those in proteoglycan. For example, calculation of the molar ratio of glucosamine$_{HA}$:

glucosamine$_{KS}$ for bovine articular cartilage (AM) from the
data of Thonar et $al.$ (1978) gives values of 0.14-0.16:1.0
throughout life.

It should be noted that not all hyaline cartilages show
similar changes in HA concentration with age. Using a specific
assay (Hatae & Makita, 1975), estimates of HA in rabbit costal
cartilage were 0.90 ± SD 0.14 mg/g dry wt for neonates (n = 5
litters), 0.76 ± 0.13 mg/g for 6-month-old rabbits (n = 9) and
1.11 ± 0.13 mg/g for 2½-year-old animals (Torabian & Mason,
1980).

INTERACTION WITH CARTILAGE PROTEOGLYCANS

Cartilage proteoglycans interact with HA to form large
proteoglycan aggregates (Hardingham & Muir, 1972; 1974;
Hascall & Heinegård, 1974a). A third component, link protein,
also interacts with the complex and appears to stabilise it
(Hascall & Sajdera, 1969; Hardingham, 1979). The experimental
evidence for the specificity and stoichiometry of the interaction have been reviewed (Hascall, 1977) and only those
features of HA structure on which it depends will be mentioned
here. Isomers of HA differing in hexosaminyl C_4 configuration
(chondroitin) or in having $\alpha 1 \rightarrow 4$ linked hexosaminyl residues
(an intermediate in heparin biosynthesis) cannot replace HA
in the interaction (Hascall & Heinegård, 1974b; Lindahl & Hook,
1978). Interaction occurs between proteoglycan monomers and HA-
oligosaccharides of decasaccharide size and larger (Hardingham
& Muir, 1973; Hascall & Heinegård, 1974b).

In an elegant series of experiments in which HA-oligomers
were modified in specific ways, Christner et $al.$ (1977, 1978,
1979a, b) have shown that to bind maximally to proteoglycan
the decasaccharide sequence must have glucuronosyl and N-
acetylglucosaminyl residues at the non-reducing and reducing
ends respectively and must contain at least one other N-acetyl
glucosamine residue, together with five unmodified carboxyl
groups in a specific spatial orientation. There is also a
requirement for glucosamine residues to be acetylated. Additional residues beyond the decasaccharide sequence, (GlcUA-
GlcNAc)$_5$, do not interact with the proteoglycan.

The interaction between HA and cartilage proteoglycan is
a strong one with a dissociation constant, K_d, of 10^{-8}-10^{-7}M
at physiological temperature and ionic strength (Nieduszynski

et al., 1980). Binding studies between either proteoglycan core-protein and HA, or between proteoglycan and HA-oligomers of decasaccharide or larger size, give association constants in agreement with this (Christer *et al.*, 1978; Cleland, 1979). Under physiological conditions most interactions between glycosaminoglycans and other macromolecules, including collagen, are electrostatic, affinity depending on charge density, molecular weight and the iduronate:glucuronate content of the polyanion (Lindahl & Höök, 1978). However, for the HA-proteoglycan interaction, the specific structural requirements for the glycosaminoglycan, the equally specific structural requirements for the proteoglycan core-protein (Hardingham *et al.*, 1976) and the high dissociation constant, point to a more complex association with multiple specific points of attachment between the two molecules. The tightness of the binding is considerably greater than that reported for lectin-carbohydrate ligand associations, K_a, 10^{-2}-10^{-4}M (Goldstein & Hayes, 1978).

Until recently it was believed that aggregation occurred only between hyaluronic acid and cartilage specific proteoglycans. In cartilage its role appears to be to organise the monomer proteoglycan into stable immobilised structures filling the interstices of the collagen network extending through the matrix. The entrapment creates a high internal osmotic pressure and consequently water is retained in the matrix giving the tissue its characteristic turgor (Rees, 1975). In articular cartilage, compression causes intramolecular reactions within the structure to increase and solvent is displaced from the proteoglycan molecular domain. The reverse occurs when the compressing force is removed (Hascall, 1977). These molecular characteristics give articular cartilage its resiliance, deformability under load, and return to original shape on decompression.

Proteoglycans from intervertebral disc also form aggregates with HA (Stevens *et al.*, 1979), presumably conferring similar physiological properties on this cartilage-like tissue, as in articular cartilage. Recently, however, it has been found that proteoglycans from several non-cartilagenous tissues and cells, of diverse origin, also form aggregates with hyaluronate. For example a chondroitin sulphate-proteoglycan from glial cells (Norling *et al.*, 1978) and a chondroitin-dermatan sulphate-proteoglycan from aorta (McMurtrey *et al.*, Oegema *et al.*, 1979) both form aggregates. In contrast a chondroitin sulphate-proteoglycan from skin (Dante *et al.*, 1979) and a dermatan sulphate-proteoglycan from follicular fluid (Yanagishita *et al.*, 1979) do not interact with hyaluronate.

Although *in vitro* demonstration of HA-proteoglycan interaction does not prove, *per se*, that the phenomenon occurs *in vivo*, these recent reports lead to the speculation that proteoglycan aggregates may have far wider physiological importance in a number of specific tissues than was higherto suspected.

The proximity of neighbouring decassacharide sequences to which proteoglycans are bound on HA will depend on two factors. First the glycosaminoglycan chains of adjacent proteoglycans cannot occupy the same space (Comper & Laurent, 1978) and their length therefore determines the minimum distance between adjacently bound molecules. For example, proteoglycans having chondroitin sulphate chains 30 disaccharide units in length could not occupy binding sites on hyaluronic acid closer than 60 disaccharide units apart. This was confirmed by electron microscopy (Rosenberg *et al.*, 1975). Secondly, the concentration of HA, or the number of available HA-binding sites, relative to the number of proteoglyan molecules will determine whether the latter are bound in close or distant proximity to one another. When saturating amounts of proteoglycan are present, the size of the aggregate formed will be related to the length of the HA chain.

The size of the aggregate may have physiological significance. Long bones grow by formation of a cartilagenous matrix in the epiphyseal plates, calcification of the matrix and finally replacement of the calcified tissue by bone. Ultramicrocentrifugation studies on extracellular matrix fluid samples from the cartilagenous plate have demonstrated the presence of large proteoglycan-aggregates which inhibit mineral growth *in vitro* in a synthetic lymph seeded with a mineral phase (Cuervo *et al.*, 1973). When they are selectively removed, mineral growth proceeds, despite the presence of smaller proteoglycan-aggregates in the lymph. Thus, the size of the aggregates present may be an important factor in regulating the onset of calcification in the epiphyseal cartilage.

Studies on rachitic rats (in which epiphyseal calcification is inhibited) and on animals recovering from rickets (calcification resumes) suggest changes in aggregate size occur during calcification *in vivo*. Weight average sedimentation coefficients for the total proteoglycan population in cartilage fluid samples fell from 65s to 55s during healing (Pita *et al.*, 1979). By computing differential g(s) distribution functions from the sedimentation data, the investigators were able to distinguish three subpopulations of proteoglycans in rachitic cartilage fluid - monomeric proteoglycans (0-32s), large aggregates (63-165s) and an intermediate population (35-60s). Although the latter probably includes some large monomers, and possibly dimers (Sheehan *et al.*, 1978), it seems likely that it also contains small aggregates. It is tempting to speculate that the onset of calcification is accompanied by a shift from large aggregates to smaller ones.

Recent evidence indicates that HA-proteoglycan interaction occurs outside the cell soon after secretion and rapidly becomes irreversible when link protein binds to the complex (Kimura *et al.*, 1979; Hardingham, 1979). If large aggregates in epiphyseal cartilage have a similar stability, changes in aggregate size prior to calcification are unlikely to arise from their partial dissociation to small aggregates in the matrix. Pita *et al.* (1979) have proposed that the two populations of proteoglycan-aggregate could be due to two different populations of HA (presumably of different chain length), or alternatively, to temporal changes in the relative proportion of HA and proteoglycan synthesised. If this is so, a shift toward smaller aggregates just prior to calcification would require chondrocytes to switch synthesis in favour of shorter HA chains or to increase HA synthesis relative to proteoglycan synthesis, whilst maintaining turnover of existing matrix components. There is good electron microscopic evidence to show that strands of HA from bovine articular and nasal cartilage and chick epiphyseal cartilage vary in length between 400-4000 nm (Rosenberg *et al.*, 1975; Kimura *et al.*, 1978). Sweet *et al.* (1979) have suggested that some HA strands in bovine articular cartilage are so short **as** to only accommodate the binding of one or a few proteoglycan molecules. There is no information available on whether chondrocytes can switch selectively from synthesis of a long form of the polymer to a short form. With respect to changing HA concentrations in the tissue, evidence suggesting an increase towards the calcifying zone has been cited above.

An alternative hypothesis explaining the presence of two aggregate populations in epiphyseal cartilage is that smaller aggregates are derived from larger ones. An obvious mechanism for this would be by limited endoglycosidase cleavage of the

HA chain of the intact aggregate, but there is no evidence so far for the existance of a hyaluronidase in cartilage (Lust & Pronsky, 1972; Bollet & Nance, 1966). Mammalian lysozyme, an enzyme found in cartilage as well as other tissues, can, however, reduce the average sediemntation coefficient of epiphyseal cartilage fluid proteoglycans *in vitro* when incubated with them at very high concentrations (Kuettner *et al.*, 1974). It appears to do so by bringing about a reduction in large aggregates and an increase in the monomer and intermediate proteoglycan populations (Pita *et al.*, 1975). It does not appear to have hyaluronidase activity (Greenwald, 1976). Further investigation is therefore required to elucidate the mechanism of its action and particularly whether it modifies one of the components of proteoglycan-aggregate by binding specifically to it.

INTERACTION WITH CARTILAGE LINK PROTEIN

A *stable* proteoglycan-aggregate consists of three components, hyaluronic acid, proteoglycan and link proteins. There are two major link proteins, mol. wt. about 40,000 and 50,000 (Keiser *et al.*, 1972; Hascall & Heinegård, 1974a). A third minor link protein has been identified by high resolution techniques (Baker & Caterson, 1977). They are structurally similar, differences in molecular weight probably being due to carbohydrate composition (Baker & Caterson, 1979). Only a single link protein is present in the proteoglycan-aggretes isolated from some cartilages (De Luca *et al.*, 1977; Oegema *et al.*, 1975).

Hardingham (1979) has shown that aggregates containing link protein are more stable at neutral pH, at temperatures up to 50°C and in urea than link-free aggregates. Moreover, HA-oligosaccharides could compete for and displace proteoglycan from link-free aggregates but not from link-stablised ones. *In vitro* studies with chondrocyte cultures demonstrated that link-stabilised aggregates are formed outside the cell (Kimura *et al.*, 1979). Within 2 hours after synthesis, 70% of the aggregate formed was link-stablised.

Link protein may have separate binding sites for proteoglycan and HA. Purified ^{14}C-labelled link protein cosediments and cochromatographs with proteoglycan in the absence of HA (Caterson & Baker, 1978). A similar experiment with ^{14}C-link protein and HA was less successful in demonstrating an association between these components as recoveries of the protein were low and sedimentation profiles poorly matched. However, Hascall & Heinegård (1974b) were able to show that link protein from bovine nasal cartilage cochromatographed with HA on Sepharose 2B. Both major link proteins bound HA. At low HA to protein ratios the glycosaminoglycan was probably saturated with protein, which resulted in coalescence between HA molecules. It is significant in this respect that link protein contains a high proportion of hydrophobic amino acids (Baker & Caterson, 1979). Oegema *et al.* (1977) have confirmed that link protein from Swarm rat chondrosarcoma also co-chromatographs with HA on Sepharose 2B.

Nothing is currently known about the chemical mechanism or binding constants for the link protein interactions with HA and proteoglycan. In chondrocyte cultures, proteoglycans are probably secreted as monomers and form reversible aggregates with HA outside the cell. Link protein then interacts and irreversibly "locks" the proteoglycan on to the HA (Kimura *et al.*, 1979). Experiments in which the HA-binding region of proteoglycan was dansylated under different conditions indicate that it has separate binding sites for HA and link protein (Heinegård & Hascall, 1979). It remains to be determined whether link protein binds both the proteoglycan HA-binding region site and HA at the same time, in aggregates formed *in vivo*.

Various proposals have been made about the significance of the link protein interactions. Link protein may modify the conformation of the HA-binding region to favour its stable association with HA (Caterson & Baker, 1978), enhance immobilisation of proteoglycans within the fibrous meshwork of the extracellular matrix by the "locking" effect or protect proteoglycan aggregates from random proteolytic degradation (Hardingham, 1979). It may also modify the overall shape and fluidity of the proteoglycan aggregate, thus contibuting to the formation of an ordered supramolecular architecture outside the cell.

INTERACTION WITH FIBRONECTIN

Fibronectin functions as an adhesive protein, binding cells together or to a collagen substratum (Yamada & Olden, 1978). It is not synthesised by chondrocytes surrounded by a matrix but is made when the matrix is absent (Dessau *et al.*,

1978). It may therefore be an important extracellular component during the early development of cartilage matrix.

Jilek & Hörmann (1979) have found that heparin promotes
the interaction of fibronectin with native type III, and to
a lesser degree, type I collagen. Heparin may act by cata-
lysing the conversion of globular fibronectin to a filamentous form which has greater affinity for the collagen.
Surprisingly, hyaluronic acid inhibits the precipitation of
soluble native collagen when it is mixed with fibronectin-
heparin. It was proposed that the HA interferes with the
interaction between the collagen and modified fibronectin.

Chondrocytes normally synthesise type II collagen, except when seeded in low density monolayers when they switch
to type I (Muller *et al.*, 1977), or are subcultured, when
they produce type I and III collagen (Benya *et al.*, 1977).
In this respect their collagen gene expression resembles that
of less well differentiated chondrocyte precursor cells. HA
may therefore have a role to play in the interactions between
collagens and fibronectin when cartilagenous tissues differ-
entiate *in vivo*.

Some evidence has been reported to show that fibronectin
interacts with sulphated proteoglycans on the cell surface
(Perkins, 1979). In addition, it was suggested that fibronectin interacts directly or indirectly with cell surface HA
and prevents it from being removed subsequently when the cells
are washed with buffered saline. Hahn & Olden (1979) have
reported that fibronectin has a specific high affinity binding
site for HA in addition to specific sites for heparin and
collagen.

HA does not bind to collagen under physiological conditions (Lindahl & Höök, 1978).

PERICELLULAR AND CELL SURFACE HYALURONIC ACID

Histochemical investigations, transmission and scanning
electron microscopy can distinguish three components in cartilage matrix (Schenk, 1978) - a perilacunar (or pericellular)
matrix which is rich in proteoglycans, beyond which lies a
territorial matrix and yet further from the cell, an interterritorial matrix. Anderson & Sajdera (1971) treated bovine
nasal cartilage with 4M-guanidine chloride and found that 15%

of the proteoglycans were not extractable. Histological
studies showed that the residual basophilia was located exclusively in the pericellular matrix closest to the cells.
Larsson *et al.* (1973) identified HA as a component of the
unextractable glycosaminoglycans of both bovine nasal and
epiphyseal cartilage. More recently Wusteman & Gillard (1977)
found that the residual glycosaminoglycans in several hyaline
and elastic cartilages were highly enriched in HA, compared
to the tissue fraction solubilised with 4M-guanidine hydrochloride. Thus, the pericellular matrix has different properties to other parts of the extracellular matrix and is enriched in HA. Whatever other functions the pericellular
matrix may have, molecules secreted by the cell which subsequently become located in the territorial and interterritorial
matrix must pass through this region. The nature and arrangement of macromolecules in the pericellular matrix must therefore influence the type and rate of diffusion of other molecules through it.

HA is associated with the cell surface of several types
of cultured cells (Fraser *et al.*, 1970; Sato *et al.*, 1977;
Underhill & Dorfman, 1978). Mikuni-Takagaki and Toole (1980)
have proposed that cell adherence to the substratum may involve both strong and weak interactions, the latter involving
surface HA and occurring during periods of relative instability
in the cell's life, such as during mitosis, cell movement, or
following transformation. Little is known, however, about the
association of endogenous HA with normal chondrocyte cell
membranes.

Transformation of chick embryo chondrocytes by Rous sarcoma virus produces cells with a more fibroblastic appearance
which synthesise more HA (Okayama *et al.*, 1977) and less
chondroitin sulphate (Muto *et al.*, 1977) than controls. The
newly synthesised HA is secreted from the transformed cells
and passes rapidly through a cell layer-associated fraction
and into the medium (Mikuni-Takagaki & Toole, 1979). Neither
HA nor proteoglycan accumulate in a matrix. Nevertheless, at
any given time, a fraction of the HA may be located between
the transformed cell surface and the substratum and be involved in an interaction between them (Mikuni-Takagaki &
Toole, 1980).

At the present time similar information about the properties of HA secreted by normal chondrocytes is not available
and its possible role in interactions between the cell and

surrounding matrix or substratum, *in vivo* or *in vitro*, is unknown.

REGULATION OF PROTEOGLYCAN SYNTHESIS BY HA

Nevo & Dorfman (1972) reported that 200 μg/ml HA added to suspension cultures of chick embryo epiphyseal chondrocytes inhibited incorporation of ^{35}S-sulphate into proteoglycans by about 30%. Wiebkin & Muir (1973) found that even lower concentrations of HA (5 x 10^{-2} μg/ml) brought about a 50% inhibition of ^{35}S incorporation into proteoglycans synthesised by pig laryngeal chondrocytes in suspension culture. The inhibitory effect was specific for chondrocytes. Moreover, at higher concentrations of exogenous HA (>1.0 μg/ml) they observed that a greater proportion of the proteoglycan synthesised was retained in the cell fraction compared to controls. Monolayers of chick embryo sternal chondrocytes also showed depressed proteoglycan synthesis when treated with 20 μg/ml HA if serum was omitted from the culture medium (Solursh *et al.*, 1974). There was no effect on leucine or thymidine incorporation or on sulphate uptake, matrix turnover or collagen synthesis. The inhibition was only brought about by HA or HA-oligosaccharides. In contrast to the results obtained with suspension cultures, a high proportion of the proteoglycan synthesised by the monolayer cultures treated with HA was found in the medium. This was probably the result of the added HA binding newly secreted proteoglycan and thus competing with the formation of link-stabilised aggregates in the pericellular matrix (Solursh *et al.*, 1980; Kimura *et al.*, 1979).

Handley & Lowther (1976) incubated high density chondrocyte cultures with HA and benzyl-β-D-xyloside, an exogenous initiator of glycosaminoglycan chain synthesis, and were able to show that the inhibitory effect of HA was on proteoglycan core-protein synthesis or xylosyl transferase rather than on chondroitin sulphate synthesis. Since HA did not affect total protein synthesis they concluded that if core protein synthesis was inhibited, the effect was highly specific.

Wiebkin *et al.* (1975) found that exogenous ^{14}C-HA bound to the chondrocyte membrane and suggested that the receptor may be a proteoglycan. Subsequently it was discovered that even oligosaccharides as small as HA$_4$ could inhibit proteoglycan synthesis by chick embryo limb chondrocytes (Solursh *et al.*, 1980). Thus the receptor mechanism cannot be the same as for cartilage proteoglycan-HA interactions, since HA_{10} is the smallest oligosaccharide able to take part in this (see above). Handley & Lowther (1976) have speculated that when a highly specific membrane receptor interacts with HA, an intracellular effector is released to mediate the inhibitory action on proteoglycan synthesis. However, further investigation is required to establish the mechanism of inhibition and also the reason for the widely differing dose-response curves observed for different chondrocytes under different culture conditions. It is noteworthy that at least one chondrocyte, that from Swarm rat chondrosarcoma, does not show depressed proteoglycan synthesis in response to exogenous HA (Solursh et al., 1980).

CONTROL OF CHONDROGENESIS BY HA

Toole and Gross (1971) used the regeneration of newt limbs after amputation to study chemical changes during chondrogenesis. In the early stages when a dedifferentiated mesenchymatous blastema forms, HA synthesis was prominant. It reached maximal levels by 10 days and thereafter decreased steeply. The decrease was associated with a rise in hyaluronidase levels. Histologically, the formation of precartilage (13-20 days) correlated with the decreasing HA levels. A similar pattern of HA production followed by HA destruction was found during chondrogenesis in the devloping chick limb and axial skeleton (Toole, 1972).

Toole et al. (1972) proceeded to investigate the effect of HA on chondrogenesis in vitro. As little as 1 ng/ml HA inhibited the formation of colonies and cartilage nodules from embryonic chick somites and limb buds in culture. They proposed that HA interferes with the differentiation of mesenchymal cells, preventing their aggregation and facilitating their diffusion, and that removal of HA by hyaluronidase reverses these effects. Thyroxine, growth hormone and calcitonin, all of wbich stimulate production of cAMP, as well as cAMP itself, prevent the HA inhibitory effects on chick somite cells (Toole, 1973).

It has been suggested (Toole et al., 1972) that the effect of HA on cell aggregation may lead to alteration in the rates of synthesis of specific differentiated cell products like chondroitin sulphate/keratan sulphate proteoglycan. If this is so, it poses the question as to whether the mechanism

of repression is the same as that by which proteoglycan synthesis in differentiated chondrocytes is inhibited by HA.

HA may have other roles in embryonic development in
addition to regulating the onset of chondrogenesis (Manasek,
1975; Toole, 1976; Solursh et al., 1979).

BIOSYNTHESIS AND TURNOVER OF HA IN CARTILAGE

The cell free synthesis of HA has been investigated with
cell fractions obtained from Group A Streptococci (Markovitz
et al., 1959; Sugahara et al., 1979), rat fibrosarcoma
(Hopwood et al., 1974) and human skin fibroblasts from normal
persons and Marfan syndrome patients (Appel et al., 1979).
In all cases the HA-synthetase activity was located in the
high speed membrane fraction (100,000 x g fraction). It is
generally accepted that chain elongation proceeds by alternate addition of monosaccharides from UDP-glucuronic acid and
UDP-N acetylglucosamine to the nascent chain, though Sugahara
et al. (1979) have drawn attention to the fact that the available experimental evidence does not eliminate the possible
participation of a disaccharide unit intermediate in the process. ATP is required for the cell free synthesis of HA by
fractions from fibroblasts (Hopwood et al., 1974; Osterlin &
Jacobsen, 1968; Appel et al., 1979). Its presence may help
to preserve levels of UDP-N acetylglucosamine by competing
for phosphatases in the membrane (Appel et al., 1979). In
the streptococcal system pulse-chase experiments have shown
that the growing chain is attached to the membrane and is
only released on completion (Sugahara, 1979). The factors
which determine HA-chain termination are unknown.

The mechanism of initiation of HA synthesis is also unknown, though it is of great interest since it may be a key
point for regulation of the process. Several alternative
initiation mechanisms must be considered, including the involvement of a core-protein, a monosaccharide or oligosaccharide acceptor, or a lipid intermediate in the process.

Many highly purified preparations of HA are associated
with small amounts of protein (see Sugahara et al., 1979 for
refs) including HA isolated from cartilage (Cleland & Sherblom,
1977). It has been proposed that the protein is a covalently
linked core-protein (Scher & Hamerman, 1972) but other investigations have shown that protein can bind non-specifically to

HA (Niedermeier & Gramling, 1970). Varma *et al.* (1974, 1975)
failed to find alkali-labile O-glycosidic linkages to serine
or threonine in protein associated with HA, demonstraing that
if a covalent link exists, it is unlike that between chondroitin
sulphate and core protein (Rodén & Schwartz, 1975).

Several investigators have studied the effect of protein
synthesis inhibitors on HA synthesis in cell or organ cultures
and different results have been recorded. Kleine (1978) for
example, incubated slices of calf rib cartilage with puromyein
or cycloheximide over a period of 90 min and reported that HA
synthesis was stimulated, whilst proteoglycan synthesis was
inhibited. In primary cultures of chondrocytes from rat
chondrosarcoma, cycloheximide stimulated HA-synthesis during
the first 45 min of incubation, but thereafter progressive
inhibition occurred so that by 225 min, HA production was only
about 33% of controls. Proteoglycan synthesis was similarly
inhibited (Mason *et al.*, 1980).

HA synthesis by cells other than chondrocytes is inhibited
to varying degrees by puromycin and cycloheximide. Skin fibroblasts from normal children and Hurler syndrome patients
(Matalon & Dorfman, 1968) and from normal human and Marfan
patients (Lemberg & Dorfman, 1973) decrease HA synthesis in
response to protein inhibition by these agents. Similarly,
Smith *et al.* (1968) observed considerable decreases in HA
synthesis by normal and rheumatoid synovial cells and by mouse
3T6 cells when treated with the inhibitors. It is noteworthy,
however, that small increases in HA synthesis by synovial cells
were recorded during the first 6 hours of the cycloheximide
block.

Differences in the degree of inhibition of HA synthesis
in the same cell type, for example, skin fibroblasts (Matalon
& Dorfman, 1968; Lemberg & Dorfman, 1973) may result from the
different inhibitor concentrations used in different experiments. The degree of inhibition of proteoglycan synthesis in
chondrocytes is sensitive to quite small changes in low concentrations of cycloheximide (Kato *et al.*, 1978).

Other factors must be considered in seeking an explanation for the initial stimulation, and then inhibition, of
HA synthesis during inhibition of protein synthesis. 75% of
the UDP-N-acetylhexosamine in neonatal rat epiphyseal cartilage is utilised for glycoprotein synthesis and 25% for glycosaminoglycans, of which HA constitutes only about 4% (Handley
& Phelps, 1972). Thus the 2-3 fold increase in the UDP-N-
acetylhexosamine pool in chondrocytes during cycloheximide

block (Telser *et al.*, 1965) is consistent with a dramatic decrease in utilisation of the nucleotide for glycoprotein synthesis and occurs even though UDP-N-acetylglucosamine is a feed-
back inhibitor of glucosamine synthetase (Kornfeld *et al.*,
1964) on its own biosynthetic pathway. The enzyme is under
complex control (Winterburn & Phelps, 1971a,b) and, although
already partly inhibited in neonatal cartilage in the steady
state (Handley & Phelps, 1972), does not appear to be totally
suppressible in these conditions.

The failure to shut off UDP-N-acetylhexosamine synthesis
when protein synthesis is inhibited is important since increases in its pool size (up to 30 nmoles/mg tissue) stimulate
synthesis of both chondroitin sulphate and HA by chondrocytes
(Kim & Conrad, 1974). Such increases can be induced by rais-
ing the concentration of D-glucosamine to 2.0 mM in the culture medium. Further increases do not increase the nucleotide
pool size but inhibit chondroitin sulphate synthesis, probably
as a consequence of inhibiting protein, and therefore core
protein synthesis. In contrast, HA synthesis continues to be
stimulated up to 25 mM D-glucosamine (Kim & Conrad, 1974).

Thus, following protein synthesis inhibition, partially
glycosylated glycoproteins will be completed rapidly, after
which the UDP-N-acetylhexosamine pool will increase in size.
Further synthesis of proteoglycan core protein must also be
inhibited, so chondroitin sulphate synthesis would continue
only until those chains initiated before the block were completed. The observation that chondroitin sulphate synthesis
is stimulated by increased intracellular levels of UDP-N-
acetylglucosamine suggests that the UDP-glucuronic acid pool,
normally rate limiting in glycosaminoglucuronan synthesis
(Handley & Phelps, 1972), must also change when the steady
state condition of the tissue is disturbed (Gainey & Phelps,
1972).

The limited evidence relating to HA synthesis suggests
that it can continue at an enhanced rate for some time (e.g.
Kliene, 1978) after protein inhibition starts before it is
inhibited itself (p. 15). Several factors could contribute
to this. First, completed HA chains may be up to 50 times,
or more, longer than chondroitin sulphate chains. Thus, incomplete HA chains would, on average, take longer to complete
than incomplete chondroitin sulphate chains following the
blockade, assuming synthesis of each is equally stimulated.
Secondly, HA synthesis may be initiated on a non-protein
acceptor, in which case it would continue for a period dependent on the half-life of the HA synthetase. In the hybrid B6

cell line the synthetase has a half-life of only 2-3.5 hours
(Tomida *et al.*, 1974) but this may not be typical of all cells.
A third speculation is that if protein acceptor is involved, a
large pool of it may be available in the cell for glycosylation
after protein synthesis is inhibited. Moreover, if a protein
acceptor is utilised, it is possible that it may not remain
with the HA after chain termination. Another glycosaminoglycan, Heparin, is synthesised as a proteoglycan but is
usually found as free single polysaccharide chains as a result
of concerted enzyme action on the proteoglycan following its
synthesis (Robinson *et al.*, 1978).

There are examples of polysaccharide synthesis in which
chain initiation is carried out by transfer of a sugar from
its nucleotide to another saccharide. Glycogen is normally
synthesised by addition of glucose units to existing glycogen
primers but synthesis can be initiated with maltose as primer
(Goldemberg, 1962). In the mammary gland lactose is syn-
thetised by transfer of galactose from its UDP-derivative to
glucose. The galactosyl transferase is normally involved in
glycoprotein synthesis but its action is modified to use glucose as an acceptor by the "specifier protein" α-lactalbumin
(Ginsburg & Stadtman, 1970). Lactose itself may then serve
as an acceptor for other transferases in the synthesis of
milk oligosaccharides (Kobata *et al.*, 1978). Rodén and
Schwartz (1975) have drawn attention to the observation that
in the initiation of chondroitin sulphate synthesis, galactosyl transferase I can function *in vitro* with D-xylose as an
acceptor and is therefore one of the few glycosyltransferases
which can utilise a monosaccharide for this.

The possible involvement of a mono-, or oligosaccharide,
acceptor in the initiation of HA synthesis should be considered. Sugahara *et al.* (1979) found a low molecular weight
(MW 1100) component was produced by the streptococcal cell-
free HA synthesising system. It was labelled with $[^{14}C]$
glucuronic acid and probably also contained N-acetylglucosamine. Radioactivity could not be transferred from it to HA
in the experimental system used, so no conclusion regarding
its role was reached. A variety of added sugars, glycosides,
HA-trisaccharide and pentasaccharide and HA itself failed to
stimulate HA synthesis in cell-free systems from strepto-
coccus, rat fibrosarcoma (Sugahara *et al.*, 1979) and normal
and Marfan skin fibroblasts (Appel *et al.*, 1979). Lemberg
(1978) has reported that synthesis was promoted by added HA
in Marfan skin fibroblast cultures. It is unlikely that the
exogenous HA could act as a primer in these circumstances and
the result suggests the effect may be mediated via an interaction with the cell membrane.

Several recent investigations have given attention to the possible role of lipid-linked oligosaccharide intermediates in HA synthesis. Oligosaccharides linked to proteins via N-asparagine bonds are first synthesised as dolicol phosphate derivatives and then transferred from the polyisoprenoid to the protein (Waechter & Lennarz, 1976). The antibiotic, tunicamycin, specifically inhibits the formation of these lipid intermediates. A rat fibrosarcoma which was very active in synthesising HA (Hopwood *et al.*, 1974) also synthesised lipid-N-acetylglucosamine, lipid-N-acetylglucosamine-glucuronic acid, and lipid tetra- and hexasaccharides with the same disaccharide unit (Hopwood & Dorfman, 1977). However, tunicamycin had no inhibitory effect on HA synthesis by the fibrosarcoma (Appel *et al.*, 1979), suggesting that the lipid oligosaccharides were not precursors of the polysaccharide.

Although Takatsuki *et al.* (1977) found that tunicamycin inhibited all glycosaminoglycan synthesis by chick embryo fibroblasts, all other investigations so far support the proposal that dolichol intermediates are not involved in HA synthesis. Thus, tunicamycin did not inhibit formation of the polysaccharide in embryonic chick fibroblasts (Hart & Lennarz, 1978), cultured rat glial cells (Sugahara *et al.*, 1979) or in the streptococcal system (Sugahara *et al.*, 1979).

There is little information available on the turnover of HA in cartilage. Handley & Phelps (1972) calculated the turnover rates of the glycosaminoglycans in neonatal rat epiphyseal cartilage. HA turned over in about 120 hours and chondroitin sulphate in 70 hours. Gillard *et al.* (1975) measured the specific activities of HA and chondroitin sulphate after incubating articular cartilage slices in [^{14}C]acetate. The specific activity of HA was considerably higher than that of chondroitin sulphate, suggesting that HA turned over more rapidly. Kleine & Stephan (1976) followed the time-course of specific labelling of HA and chondroitin sulphate in calf rib cartilage. The HA pool had lower specific activity than the chondroitin sulphate pool except after very short incubation times, when it was higher. Further experiments need to be carried out before any conclusions can be reached about the significance of these seemingly contradictory results. The design of such experiments should take account of the potential for differential stimulation of HA and chondroitin sulphate synthesis when glucosamine is added to the medium (Kim & Conrad, 1974).

HA SYNTHESIS BY SWARM RAT CHONDROSARCOMA CHONDROCYTES IN
PRIMARY CULTURE

The preceding review has attempted to draw attention to
the importance of HA as both a structural and regulatory molecule in cartilage and to the fact that despite numerous investigations on this and other tissues, many questions still
remain to be answered regarding the mechanism of its synthesis,
export from the cell, metabolic turnover and physiological
function. The remainder of this paper describes, in summary,
a system for the study of HA synthesis by chondrocytes in
tissue culture.

Chondrocytes from the Swarm rat chondrosarcoma (Choi *et
al*, 1971) were used. Recent studies have resulted in a detailed knowledge of the structure of the proteoglycans
(Oegema *et al*., 1975), proteoglycan aggregates (Faltz *et al*.,
1979a,b), link protein (Oegema *et al*., 1977) and collagen
(Smith *et al*., 1975; Breitkreutz *et al*., 1979) produced by
the chondrosarcoma. The proteoglycans do not contain keratan
sulphate but in every other respect the macromolecular products of the tumour appear to be typical of those synthesised
by chondrocytes in normal cartilage. The biosynthesis of proteoglycans by chondrocytes isolated from the tumour and kept
in primary tissue culture has also been investigated (Kimura
et al., 1979). Thus, a great deal is already known about the
major extracellular components made by these cells and this,
together with the large number of chondrocytes which can be
obtained from the tumour (approximately 10^7 cells/g wet weight),
suggested it may be a suitable tissue for the investigation
of HA synthesis by chondrocytes.

Primary cell cultures were prepared as described by
Kimura *et al*. (1979). Briefly, small pieces of chondrosarcoma
tissue were pressed through a 1 mm sieve and then homogenised
at low speed. Then, following digestion with trypsin and
collagenase, single chondrocytes were obtained by filtering
the cell suspension through a 70μ screen and next, a 20μ
screen. The cells were plated at high density (e.g. 6 x 10^6
cells/60 mm dish) on plastic tissue culture dishes and maintained in Dulbecco's modified Eagle's medium (MEM) containing
organic buffers and 20% foetal calf serum (FCS). Under these
conditions the chondrocytes form a layer on the dish about
three cells deep and an extracellular matrix is established
between them. The cultures were labelled with D-[$6-^3$H]-glucos-
amine HCl or   L-[$3-^3$H]serine, with or without [^{35}S]sulphate.
Total incorporation of the isotopes into proteoglycans and
other molecules was estimated by chromatography of tissue

culture fractions on prepacked Sephadex G-25 columns (Lohmander
et al., 1979). When labelled with 50 µCi ^{3}H-glucosamine/ml
in Dulbecco's MEM + 20% FCS on day 2 or day 3 in culture, the
chondrocytes, typically, incorporate about 2.8 x 10^5 dpm/h/10^6
cells into macromolecules. The amount of glucosamine (specific
activity 38 Ci/mmol) added to the medium was small and no
stimulation of ^{35}S-proteoglycan synthesis was observed in dual
label studies compared to controls in which only ^{35}S was
present.

^{3}H-HA and ^{3}H, ^{35}S-glycosaminoglycans in tissue culture
fractions were measured by a procedure based on the following
steps: (a) removal of unincorporated isotope by Sephadex G-25
chromatography, (b) papain digestion, (c) dialysis and concentration by freeze-drying (d) digestion with chondroitinase
ABC (Saito *et al.*, 1968), (e) thin layer chromatography on
precoated cellulose plates to separate the unsaturated di-
saccharides of chondroitin-6-sulphate, chondroitin-4-sulphate,
chondroitin and HA, released by the enzyme, (f) extraction of
the spots with 0.5M-HCl and counting for radioactivity. Car-
rier glycosaminoglycans were added at the beginning of the
procedure and the recovery of ^{35}S-glycosaminoglycans was
greater than 90%. About 40% of the total ^{3}H-glucosamine incorporated into macromolecules was lost during the dialysis
step and this was shown to be due to loss of glycopeptides
generated by the action of papain on glycoproteins. Recovery
of ^{3}H-glycosaminoglycans was of the same order as ^{35}S-
glycosaminoglycans. The conditions adopted for the chondroitinase ABC digestion (0.002 units enzyme/µg chondroitin sulphate,
Tris-acetate buffer, pH 8.0) ensured complete degradation of
^{3}H-HA in the presence of chondroitin sulphate. Fluoride was
included in the buffer to inhibit any traces of sulphatase
activity which could contaminate the enzyme preparation
(Handley & Lowther, 1979).

Using the chondroitinase ABC method it was found that ^{3}H-
HA synthesis accounted for 11.6% ± 2.0(± SD, n=7) of the total
^{3}H-glycosaminoglycans synthesised when 2 day cultures were
labelled over a 6 hour period. The ^{3}H-disaccharide ratios
for Δdi-6-S:Δdi-4-S:Δdi-O-S:Δdi-HA in the medium of such cultures were, typically, 0.06:1.00:0.20:0.16. Further experiments in which the cell cultures were labelled continuously
for 2, 6, 12 or 24 hours, showed that the incorporation of
^{35}S-sulphate into proteoglycans and of ^{3}H-glucosamine into
the glycosaminoglycans followed a linear course through 24
hours. The proportion of ^{3}H-HA to total ^{3}H-glycosaminoglycan
synthesised remained more or less constant during the experiment with a mean value of 12.5%.

Experiments were carried out to determine how the newly synthesised molecules were distributed in the culture. After the labelling period, the medium was removed and the cell layer and associated matrix extracted with 4.0M-guanidine HCl containing a proteinase inhibitor cocktail, for 1 hour, at 4°C. The extract was removed and the cell residue solubilised with 0.5M-NaOH or by papain digestion. In a representative experiment in which cell cultures were labelled on day 3 in culture for 6 hours, the distribution of ^{3}H-HA between the medium, extract and residue fractions was 61.3%, 19.4% and 19.3%, whereas that of ^{3}H-chondroitin sulphate was 57.4%, 27.8% and 14.7% respectively.

The time course of secretion of ^{3}H-HA from the cells into the matrix and on into the culture medium was compared with that of ^{35}S-proteoglycan and ^{3}H-chondroitin sulphate. Day 3 cultures (6 x 10^6 cells) were incubated with 250 µCi ^{3}H-glucosamine or 100 µCi ^{35}S-sulphate for 30 min. The medium was removed and the cell layer washed rapidly (x2) with fresh medium. The cultures were then incubated in fresh medium for various periods up to 3.0 hours and the distribution of labelled macromolecules in the pulse medium, chase medium, cell layer extract and cell residue measured. At the end of the 30 min pulse most of the ^{3}H-HA (72%) and ^{3}H-chondroitin sulphate (62%) were located in the cell residue with only small amounts (9% and 11% respectively) in the medium. After 30 min chase the amount of both molecules in the cell residue had decreased and 28% ^{3}H-HA was recovered in the cell layer extract and 33% in the medium. The corresponding figures for ^{3}H-chondroitin sulphate were 42% (extract) and 27% (medium). After a 3 hour chase, 86% of ^{3}H-HA and 68% of ^{3}H-chondroitin sulphate were found in the medium, leaving 9% and 22% respectively in the extract and the remainder associated with the cell residue. As would be expected, the ^{35}S-proteoglycan "pulse chase profile" was very similar to the ^{3}H-chondroitin sulphate profile.

The results show that most of the HA and chondroitin sulphate synthesised in a 30 min period pass quite rapidly out of the cell, through the cell-associated matrix and into the medium. Rather more of the total HA than of the total proteoglycan accumulated in the medium and appeared to do so more rapidly. If all the HA synthesised by the cell was involved in HA-proteoglycan interactions outside the cell it would be expected that both molecules would pass into the medium in the same relative proportions and at the same rate. The results, therefore, raise the question as to whether a separate pool of HA exists which is not involved in such interactions and could therefore pass more rapidly through the cell-associated matrix than HA bound in proteoglycan aggregates.

In conclusion, the preliminary results of investigations on HA synthesis by Swarm rat chondrosarcoma chondrocytes in culture suggest that the system may be a useful one for further studies in this area. It remains to be established whether the relatively large amounts of HA synthesised by the cells is typical of chondrocytes in primary tissue culture, or is related to the neoplastic origin of the cells which are in most other respects well differentiated chondrocytes.

Acknowledgement. Experimental work on the chondrosarcoma chondrocytes was carried out in collaboration with Dr. Vincent C. Hascall and Dr. James H. Kimura at the Laboratory of Biochemistry, N.I.D.R., National Institutes of Health, Bethesda, MD, U.S.A.

REFERENCES

Anderson HC, Sajdera SW (1971). J Cell Biol 49: 650-663.
Antonopoulos CA, Gardell S, Szirmai JA, De Tyssonsk ER (1964). Biochim Biophys Acta 83: 1-19.
Appel A, Horwitz AL, Dorfman A (1979). J Biol Chem 254: 12199-12203.
Baker JR, Caterson B (1977). Biochem Biophys Res Commun 77: 1-10.
Baker JR, Caterson B (1979). J Biol Chem 254: 2387-2393.
Bayliss MT, Ali SY (1978). Biochem J 176: 683-693.
Benya PD, Padilla SR, Nimni ME (1977). Biochem 16: 865-872.
Bollet AJ, Nance JL (1966). J Clin Invest 45: 1170-1177.
Breitkreutz D, Diaz de Leon L, Paglia L, Gay S, Swarm RL, Stern R (1979). Cancer Res 39: 5093-5100.
Caterson B, Baker J (1978). Biochem Biophys Res Commun 80: 496-503.
Choi HU, Meyer K, Swarm R (1971) Proc Natl Acad Sci USA 68: 877-879.
Christner JE, Brown ML, Dziewiatkowski DD (1977). Biochem J 167: 711-716.
Christner JE, Brown ML, Dziewiatkowski DD (1978). Anal Biochem 90: 22-32.
Christner JE, Brown ML, Dziewiatkowski DD (1979a). J Biol Chem 254: 4624-4630.
Christner JE, Brown ML, Dziewiatkowski DD (1979b). J Biol Chem 254: 12303-12305.
Cleland RL (1979) Biochem Biophys Res Commun 87: 1140-1145.
Cleland RL, Sherblom AP (1977). J Biol Chem 252: 420-426.

Comper WD, Laurent TC (1978). Physiol Rev 58: 255-315.
Cuervo LA, Pita JC, Howell DS (1973). Calc Tiss Res 13: 1-10.
Damle SP, Kieras FJ, Tzeng W-K, Gregory JD (1979). J Biol
   Chem 254: 1614-1620.
De Luca S, Heinegård D, Hascall VC, Kimura JH, Caplan AI (1977).
   J Biol Chem 252:6600-6608.
Dessau W, Sasse J, Timpl R, Jilek F, Von der Mark K (1978).
   J Cell Biol 79: 342-355.
Faltz LL, Redi AH, Hascall GK, Martin D, Pita JC, Hascall VC
   (1979a). J Biol Chem 254: 1375-1380.
Faltz LL, Caputo CB, Kimura JH, Schrode J, Hascall VC (1979b).
   J Biol Chem 254: 1381-1387.
Fraser JR, Clarris BJ, Kont LA (1970). Aust J Biol Sci 23:
   1297-1303.
Gainey PA, Phelps CF (1972). Biochem J 128: 215-227.
Gillard GC, Caterson B, Lowther DA (1975). Biochem J 145:
   209-213.
Ginsberg A, Stadtman ER (1970). Ann Rev Biochem 39: 429-472.
Goldemberg SH (1962). Biochim Biophys Acta 56: 357-359.
Goldstein IJ, Hayes CE (1978). Adv Carb Chem Biochem 35: 127-338.
Greenwald RA (1976). Semin Arthritis Rheum 6: 35-51.
Hahn L-HE, Olden K (1979). Int Congr Biochem Abstr 336.
Handley CJ, Lowther DA (1976). Biochim Biophys Acta 444: 69-74.
Handley CJ, Lowther DA (1979). Biochim Biophys Acta 582: 234-
   245.
Handley CJ, Phelps CF (1972). Biochem J 126: 417-432.
Hardingham TE (1979). Biochem J 177: 237-247.
Hardingham TE, Adams P (1976). Biochem J 159: 143-147.
Hardingham TE, Ewins RJF, Muir H (1976). Biochem J 157: 127-
   143.
Hardingham TE, Muir H (1972). Biochim Biophys Acta 279: 401-
   405.
Hardingham TE, Muir H (1973). Biochem J 135: 905-908.
Hardingham TE, Muir H (1974). Biochem J 139: 565-581.
Hart GW, Lennarz WJ (1978). J Biol Chem 253: 5795-5801.
Hascall VC (1977). J Supramol Struc 7: 101-120.
Hascall VC, Heinegård D (1974a). J Biol Chem 249: 4232-4241.
Hascall VC, Heinegård D (1974b). J Biol Chem 249: 4242-4249.
Hascall VC, Sajdera S (1969). J Biol Chem 244: 2384-2396.
Hatae Y, Makita A (1975). Anal Biochem 64: 30-36.
Heinegård D, Hascall VC (1979). J Biol Chem 254: 921-926.
Hjertquist S-O (1964a). Acta Soc Med Upsal 69: 83-104.
Hjertquist S-O (1964b). Acta Soc Med Upsal 69: 23-40.
Hopwood JJ, Dorfman A (1977). Biochem Biophys Res Commun 75:
   472-479.
Hopwood JJ, Fitch FW, Dorfman A (1974). Biochem Biophys Res
   Commun 61: 583-590.

Inerot S, Heinegård D, Andell L, Olsson S-E (1978) Biochem J
169: 143-156.

Jilek F, Hörmann, H (1979). Hoppe-Seyler's Z Physiol Chem
360: 597-603.

Kato Y, Koji K, Kenichiro I, Kenichiro K, Suzuki S (1978) J
Biol Chem 253: 2784-2789.

Keiser H, Shulman HJ, Sandson JI (1972). Biochem J 126: 163-
169.

Kim JJ, Conrad HE (1974). J Biol Chem 249: 3091-3097.

Kimura JH, Hardingham TE, Hascall VC, Solursh M (1979) J Biol
Chem 254: 2600-2609.

Kimura JH, Osdoby P, Caplan AI, Hascall VC (1978). J Biol
Chem 253: 4721-4729.

Kleine TO (1978). Conn Tis Res 5: 195-199.

Kleine TO, Stephan R (1976). Biochim Biophys Acta 451: 444-
456.

Kobata A, Yamashita K, Tachibana Y (1978). Meth Enz 50: 216-220.

Kornfeld S, Kornfeld R, Neufeld EF, O'Brien PJ (1964). Proc
Nat Acad Sci USA 52: 371-379.

Kuettner KE, Sorgente N, Croxen RL, Howell DS, Pita JC (1974).
Biochim Biophys Acta 372: 335-344.

Larsson S-E, Ray RD, Kuettner KE (1973). Calc Tiss Res 13:
271-285.

Lemberg SI (1978). J Invest Dermatol 71: 391-395.

Lemberg SI, Dorfman A (1973). J Clin Invest 52: 2428-2433.

Lindahl U, Höök M (1978). Ann Rev Biochem 47: 385-417.

Lohmander LS, Hascall VC, Caplan AI (1979) J Biol Chem 254:
10551-10561.

Lust G, Pronsky W (1972). Clin Chim Acta 39: 281-286.

McNicol D, Roughley PJ (1980). Biochem J 185: 705-713.

McMurtrey J, Radhakrishnamurthy B, Dalferes ER, Berenson GS,
Gregory JD (1979). J Biol Chem 254: 1621-1626.

Manasek FJ (1975). Curr Top Develop Biol 10: 35

Markovitz A, Cipondi JA, Dorfman A (1959). J Biol Chem 234:
2343-2350.

Mason RM, Kimura JH, Hascall VC (1980). Abstracts VII European Symposium on Connective Tissue Research, Prague.

Matalon R, Dorfman A (1968). Proc Nat Acad Sci USA 60: 179-185.

Mikuni-Takayaki Y, Toole BP (1979). J Biol Chem 254: 8409-8415.

Mikuni-Takayaki Y, Toole BP (1980). J Cell Biol 85: 481-488.

Muto M, Yoshimura M, Okayama M, Kaji A (1977). Proc Nat Acad
Sci USA 74: 4173-4177.

Muller PK, Lemmen C, Gay S, Gauss V, Kühn K (1977). Exp Cell
Res 108: 47-55.

Neidermeir W, Gramling E (1970). Ala J Med Sci 7: 305-309.

Nevo Z, Dorfman A (1972). Proc Nat Acad Sci USA 69: 2069-2072.

Nieduszynski IA, Sheehan JK, Phelps CF, Hardingham TE, Muir H (1980). Biochem J 185: 107-114.

Norling B, Grimelius B, Westermark B, Wasterson A (1978). Biochim Biophys Res Commun 84: 914-921.

Oegema TR, Brown M, Dziewiatkowski DD (1977) J Biol Chem 252: 6470-6477.

Oegema TR, Hascall VC, Dziewiatkowski DD (1975) J Biol Chem 250: 6151-6159.

Oegema TR, Hascall VC, Eisenstein R (1979). J Biol Chem 254: 1312-1318.

Okayama M, Yoshimura M, Muto M, Chi J, Roth S, Kaji A (1977). Cancer Res 37: 712-717.

Österlin SE, Jacobsen B (1968). Exp Eye Res 7: 497-510.

Pearson JP, Mason RM (1978). Biochem Soc Trans 6: 244-246.

Pearson JP, Mason RM (1979). Biochim Biophys Acta 583: 512-526.

Perkins ME, Ji, TH, Hynes RO (1979). Cell 16: 941-952.

Pita JC, Howell DS, Kuettner KE (1975). In Slavkin HC, Greulich RC (eds): "Extracellular Matrix Influences on Gene Expression," New York: Academic Press, p 721-726.

Pita JC, Muller FJ, Morales SM, Alarcon EJ (1979). J Biol Chem 254: 10313-10320.

Rees DA (1975). In Whelan WJ (ed): "MTP International Review of Science, Biochemistry Series 1," Vol 5 London: Butterworths, p 1-42.

Robinson HC, Horner AA, Hook M, Ogren S, Lindahl U (1978). J Biol Chem 253: 6687-6693.

Rodén L, Schwartz NB (1975). In Whelan WJ (ed) "MTP International Review of Science, Biochemistry Series 1," Vol 5, London: Butterworths, p 95-151.

Rosenberg L, Hellman W, Kleinschmidt AK (1975). J Biol Chem 250: 1877-1883.

Saito H, Yamagata T, Suzuki S (1968). J Biol Chem 243: 1536-1542.

Sato C, Kojima K, Nishizawa K (1977). Biochim Biophys Acta 470: 446-452.

Schenk RK (1978). In Weber BG, Burnner Ch, Freuler F (eds): "Die Frakturenbehandlung bei Kindern und Jugenliehen," chapter 1, Berlin: Springer-Verlag.

Scher I, Hamerman D (1972). Biochem J 126: 1073-1080.

Scott JE (1960). In Glick D (ed) "Methods of Biochemical Analysis," Vol 8, New York: Interscience Publishers Inc. p 146.

Seno M, Anno K (1960). Biochim Biophys Acta 49: 407-408.

Sheehan JK, Nieduszynski IA, Phelps CF, Muir H, Hardingham TE (1978). Biochem J 171: 109-114.

Smith C, Hamerman D (1968). Proc Soc Exp Biol Med 127: 988-991.

Smith BD, Martin GR, Miller EJ, Dorfman A (1975). Arch Biochem Biophys 166: 181-186.

Solheim K (1965). J Oslo Cy Hosp 15: 127-132.

Solheim K (1968). J Oslo Cy Hosp 18: 45-58.

Solursh M, Fisher M, Singley CT (1979) Differentiation 14: 77-84.

Solursh M, Hardingham TE, Hascall VC, Kimura JH (1980) Dev Biol 75: 121-129.

Solursh M, Vacrewyck SA, Reiter RS (1974). Dev Biol 41: 233-244.

Stevens RL, Ewins RJF, Revell PA, Muir H (1979). Biochem J 179: 561-562.

Sweet MBE, Thonar EJ-MA, Marsh J (1979). Arch Biochem Biophys 198: 439-448.

Sugahara K, Schwartz NB, Dorfman A (1979). J Biol Chem 254: 6252-6261.

Szirmai JA, De Tyssonsk EVB, Gardell S (1967). Biochim Biophys Acta 136: 331-350.

Takatsuki A, Fukui Y, Tamura G (1977). Agric Biol Chem 41: 425-427.

Telser A, Robinson HC, Dorfman A (1965). Proc Nat Acad Sci USA 54: 912-919.

Thonar EJ-MA, Sweet MBE, Immelman AR, Lyons G (1978). Calcif Tiss Res 26: 19-21.

Tomida M, Koyama H, Ono T (1974). Biochim Biophys Acta 338: 352-363.

Toole BP (1972). Develop Biol 29: 321-329.

Toole BP (1973). Science 80: 302-303.

Toole BP (1976). In Barondes SH (ed):"Neuronal Recognition," New York: Plenum Press, p 275

Toole BP, Gross J (1971). Develop Biol 26: 28-35.

Toole BP, Jackson G, Gross J (1973). Proc Nat Acad Sci USA 69: 1384-1386.

Torabian R, Mason RM (1980) Unpublished observation.

Underhill CB, Dorfman A (1978). Exp Cell Res 117: 155-164.

Varma R, Varma RS, Allen WS, Wardi AH (1974). Biochim Biophys Acta 263: 584-588.

Varma R, Varma RS, Allen WS, Wardi AH (1975). Biochim Biophys Acta 399: 139-144.

Waechter CJ, Lennarz WJ (1976). Ann Rev Biochem 45: 95-112.

Wiebkin OW, Muir H (1973). FEBS Lett 37: 42-46.

Wiebkin OW, Hardingham TE, Muir H (1975). In Slavkin HC, Greulich RC (eds): "Extracellular Matrix Influences on Gene Expression," New York: Academic Press, p 209-233.

Winterburn PJ, Phelps CF (1971a). Biochem J 121: 711-720.

Winterburn PJ, Phelps CF (1971b). Biochem J 121: 721-730.

Wusteman FS, Gillard GC (1977). Experientia 33: 721-723.

Yanagishita M, Rodbard D, Hascall VC (1979). J Biol Chem 254: 911-920.

Yamada KM, Olden K (1978). Nature 275: 179-184.

Connective Tissue Research:
Chemistry, Biology, and Physiology, Pages 113–123
© 1981 Alan R. Liss, Inc., 150 Fifth Avenue, New York, N.Y. 10011

CALCIFIABLE MATRICES

E. Bonucci

1st Institute of Pathological Anatomy,
University of Rome, Italy.

Calcifiable matrices are very numerous and virtually every organic substratum can have this property or can be converted into a calcifiable matrix under experimental or pathological conditions. Although all calcifiable matrices share the property of inducing the precipitation of inorganic substance, they can have very different chemical composition and morphological structure. Consequently, their comparative study can add many useful data to the solution of the numerous problems which are still unsolved with regard to the mechanism of the calcification process.

When an analysis of the matrices which calcify is carried out, bone is the first tissue which is usually considered. In respect to other calcifying tissues, bone is chiefly characterized by the high order of organization and degree of compactness of the collagen fibrils of its matrix. Moreover, many investigations have shown that a close relationship exists in bone matrix between the inorganic substance and the collagen periodic banding (Fitton Jackson, 1957; Dudley and Spiro, 1961; Ascenzi et al., 1965, 1967; Cooper et al., 1966; Glimcher and Krane, 1968). In particular, it has been emphasized the fact that the mineral substance, being initially deposited between a_3 and c_2 bands, that is in the area which corresponds to the so-called "hole zone" (Glimcher and Krane, 1968), induces an accentuation of the axial period of the fibrils. On the basis of these and other observations, the hypothesis has been proposed that a peculiar arrangement of chemical groups in the hole zone can induce inorganic substance deposition by a mechanism of heteroneneous nuclea-

tion followed by growth and mechanical orientation of
crystals within the collagen fibrils (Glimcher, 1959; Glimcher
and Krane, 1968).

This theory, however, does not seem to fit with all
experimental findings on calcification of bone and other
tissues. It cannot be neglected, in fact, that in areas of
initial osteogenesis the earliest crystal clusters can be
unrelated to the collagen periodic banding (Bonucci, 1971),
that the needle-shaped crystals are often placed on the
fibrils surface and in the interfibrillary space rather than
within the holes of the fibrils (Robinson and Cameron, 1956;
Ascenzi et al., 1963; Cameron, 1963; Cooper et al., 1966;
Höhling, 1969; Bonucci and De Santis, 1980), that these
crystals are often longer than the holes where they should
be located (Ascenzi et al., 1965) and that, depending on the
type of bone dealt with, not all investigations have revealed
a close relationship between mineral deposition and collagen
periodic banding (Ascenzi and Benedetti, 1959; Decker, 1966;
Bernard and Pease, 1969; Bonucci, 1971). Moreover, although
the theory referred to might be considered valid as far as
bone is concerned, it cannot be extended to those calcifying
tissues which have few collagen fibrils or none at all.

In this connection, it is convenient to make a distinc-
tion between ossification and calcification. Calcification
means deposition of mineral substance in an organic matrix,
not necessarily containing collagen fibrils; ossification
means formation and calcification of a very particular collagenous matrix, the matrix of bone. There are few doubts
that in bone the mineral substance is in some way related
to the collagen fibrils, being these structures the most
aboundant constituents of the matrix. There are even less
doubts that calcification can occur in many tissues in absence
of collagen fibrils (see, for instance, Bonucci and Sadun,
1972, 1973, 1975). If a general theory of calcification
must be found, structures other than collagen fibrils must
be taken into consideration as inductors of mineral deposition and they should be present in all the matrices which
calcify or which can be made calcifiable.

Studies with the electron microscope have shown that
an inverse relationship exists in bone between the amount of
needle-shaped crystals and the compactness of the collagen
fibrils (Bonucci, 1971). For instance, the medullary bone
of pigeons, which is characterized by relatively few collagen

fibrils in respect to an aboundant ground substance, shows
plenty of needle-shaped crystals (Bonucci and Gherardi, 1975),
having in this connection a strong similarity to the calcified
cartilage. By comparative examination of various types of
bone, the conclusion can be drawn that the lower the concentration of collagen fibrils and the greater the amount
of interfibrillary ground substance, the higher the concentration of needle-shaped crystals and the lower the amount of
mineral substance corresponding to the fibril periodic
banding. This observation leads to the conclusion that the
mineral substance in bands is probably contained within the
"holes" of the fibrils, whereas the needle-shaped crystals
are placed outside the fibrils and are related to the interfibrillary ground substance. In looking for calcification-
inducing substances it seems consequently necessary to study
the organic components which are related to the formation
of the needle-shaped crystals, which are present in all
calcifying tissues, rather than the components which lead
to the precipitation of mineral in bands, which is found
only in bone and other few compact collagenous tissues
(tendons). In the case of the needle-shaped crystals there
are few doubts that the substances which are responsible of
their formation must be components of the ground substance,
referring with this term to all non-collagenous organic
material which in connective tissues is present between the
collagen fibrils and on their surface, and in the intercellular spaces.

As far as the role of the ground substance in calcification is concerned, three types of components have chiefly
been considered, which are present in various proportion in
all the matrices which calcify: proteoglycans, lipids and
phosphoproteins.

The eventual role of proteoglycans in inducing the precipitation of mineral substance has been the object of a
relevant number of investigations and has been reviewed a
lot of times (Sobel, 1955; Cameron, 1963; Weidmann, 1963;
Urist, 1964, 1966; Bachra, 1967, 1970; Bowness, 1968; Glimcher
and Krane, 1968; Schubert and Pras, 1968; Campo, 1970;
Schiffmann et al., 1970; Bonucci, 1971; Irving, 1973). However, the matter is still reason of debate.

There is no doubt that all normal and pathological
calcifications occur in areas which contain glycoproteins
and acid proteoglycans. The role of these substances, how-

ever, is not yet completely clear, the uncertainty being increased by the fact that they are present also in tissues which do not calcify in normal conditions. The principal disagreement concerns as to whether proteoglycans promote or inhibit the calcification process. In a recent further examination of this problem, De Bernard et al. (1977) conclude that at least in calcifying cartilage glycosaminoglycans increase before calcification starts and that, afterwards, part of them are removed. It is suggested that this removal might reduce the hydrophilic power and calcium affinity of the ground substance and might break up a barrier to mineral deposition, thus allowing calcification to initiate.

Looking for the presence in calcifying cartilage of a component with calcium affinity, Vittur et al. (1972) have discovered a glycoprotein with two classes of Ca^{2+}-binding sites, which exibits also alkaline phosphatase activity (Vittur and De Bernard, 1973). The interest of this finding is obvious: by its calcium affinity on one side and by releasing or trasfering Pi on another side, this glycoprotein might play a very important role in clacium phosphate precipitation (Stagni et al., 1979). However, its precise function has not yet been determined.

The first demonstration that matrices which calcify contain lipids has been given histochemically by Irving (1963). Successively, many other investigators reached the same conclusion with histochemical, biochemical and ultrastructural methods (Irving and Wuthier, 1968; Wuthier, 1968, 1969; Shapiro, 1970; Bonucci et al., 1978).

A number of observations show that lipids, especially acidic lipids (Vogel and Boyan-Salyers, 1976), such as phosphatidylserine and phosphatidylinositol, can bind calcium and phosphorus (Irving and Wuthier, 1968) and might in this way initiate the calcification process. In line with these observations, it has been shown that complete extraction of lipids from calcified matrices can be obtained only after decalcification because of the intimate relationship lipids have with the inorganic substance (Wuthier, 1968). These results, by the way, are in agreement with findings of Bonucci (1967, 1969, 1971) which show that in calcifying areas the inorganic substance is closely connected to an organic component so that the crystals appear to be organic-inorganic structures.

The possibility that lipids play a role in calcification has been further strengthened by the discovery in rabbit long bones of calcium-acidic phospholipid-phosphate complexes (Boskey and Posner, 1976) which seem to be components of the membranes of the matrix vesicles (see below) and might be the intermediates from which needle-shaped crystals successively develop (Boskey, 1978). It is of interest that in epiphyseal cartilage the concentration of the calcium-phospholipid-phosphate complexes increases going from the reserve zone to the proliferative zone and reaches a maximum value in the hypertrophic zone, where mineralization is initiated, and a minimum value in primary spongiosa and diaphyseal bone (Boskey et al., 1980).

Other substances which are present in calcifiable matrices and can mediate or induce the onset of calcification are constituents of the ground substance. Anionic phosphoproteins have been isolated from cortical bone (Shuttleworth and Veis, 1972) and dentine (Veis et al., 1972; Di Muzio and Veis, 1978). Ca^{2+}-binding amino-acids, such as O-phosphoserine and o-phosphotreonine, have been isolated from the calcified portion of turkey leg tendonds and not from the part which does not calcify (Glimcher et al., 1979).

Another Ca^{2+}-binding amino-acid, gamma-carboxyglutamic acid, has recently been isolated from calcifying and non-calcifying matrices of various nature (Hauschka et al., 1975; Lian et al., 1976; Deyl et al., 1979; Glimcher et al., 1979; Levy et al., 1979).

From all these findings it is possible to conclude that, beside collagen fibrils, the calcifiable matrices contain a number of substances which can bind calcium and/or phosphate and which can in this way induce mineral deposition. The same substances can be found in many organic matrices which do not calcify in normal conditions; however, just owing to the presence of these substances, virtually all types of organic matrix can calcify in pathological or suitable experimental conditions. It is probably necessary and sufficient that the calcium- and phosphate-binding substances are activated either by removal of inhibitors or by interruption of the cellular control.

It cannot be neglected that the access of mineral ions to the calcifiable matrices is under cellular control and that consequently the calcification process can be promoted

or inhibited by the cellular activity. In this connection,
important new knowledge has been added by the discovery of
matrix vesicles in calcifying cartilage (Bonucci, 1967, 1970;
Anderson, 1969), bone (Bernard and Pease, 1969; Bonucci, 1971),
dentine (Bernard, 1972; Eisenmann and Glick, 1972; Slavkin
et al., 1972), and other normal and pathological tissues
(see Anderson, 1976). Matrix vesicles are membrane-bound,
extracellular bodies of cellular origin, whose matrix
possesses phosphatase activity and contains glycoproteins
and lipids and whose membrane is coated by acid proteoglycans
(see Bonucci, 1971, 1975; Anderson, 1973, 1976). The interest
of these structures is not only that of being the locus of
initial calcification in bone, cartilage, dentine and other
calcifying tissues, but also that of representing a way the
cells could exert their control on the surrounding calcifiable matrix.

In this connection, recent investigations showing that
in epiphyseal cartilage the concentration of calcium and
phosphate of matrix vesicles has an inverse correlation in
respect to that of the mitochondria (Brighton and Hunt, 1978),
suggest that the cells can exert their control by increasing
or reducing the efflux of mineral ions in the extracellular
space through variations of their intramitochondrial concentration (see also Sayegh et al., 1974).

The role of mitochondria in regulating the intracellular
concentration of calcium and phosphate is well known (see
Lehninger, 1970) and does not need to be discussed here.
Studies of pathological calcifications have shown that when
excessive intracellular concentration of mineral ions cannot
be compensated by mitochondrial activity, degeneration of the
cells follows and precipitation of calcium phosphate can
occur both within the cells themselves and in the pericellular
matrix (Bonucci and Sadun, 1973). The same phenomenon can
occur when cellular metabolic alterations inhibit the mitochondrial compensatory activity (Bonucci and De Matteis,
1968).

From all the findings which have been considered, the
following main conclusions can be drawn:
1. Calcification can occur in almost every organic matrix.
2. The efficiency of an organic matrix to induce calcification largely depends upon the presence of particular substances (in particular proteoglycans, lipids, phosphoproteins, eventually associated with collagen fibrils),

and upon the number of their active nucleating sites and the magnitude of their energy of activation.

3. The capacity of a matrix to be calcified and to some extent to become calcifiable depends upon cellular control which can promote or prevent the access of mineral ions into the matrix.

4. Pathological calcification partly depends upon disruption of this cellular control either by abnormalities of the cellular metabolic activity (dystrophic calcification) or by excessive intracellular concentration of mineral ions and consequent overstepping of the mitochondrial buffering power (metastatic calcification).

ACKNOWLEDGEMENTS

The personal investigations mentioned in this paper have been supported by grants of the Italian National Research Council.

REFERENCES

Anderson HC (1969). Vesicles associated with calcification in the matrix of epiphyseal cartilage. J Cell Biol 41:59.

Anderson HC (1973). Calcium-accumulating vesicles in the intercellular matrix of bone. In: Hard tissue growth, repair and remineralization. Elsevier-Excerpta Medica-North Holland, Amsterdam, p 213.

Anderson HC (1976). Matrix vesicles of cartilage and bone. In Bourne GH (ed): "The biochemistry and physiology of bone", Academic Press, New York, p 135.

Ascenzi A, Benedetti EL (1959). An electron microscopic study of the foetal membranous ossification. Acta Anat 37:370.

Ascenzi A, Bonucci E, Steve Bocciarelli D (1965). An electron microscope study of osteon calcification. J Ultrastruct Res 12:287.

Ascenzi A, Bonucci E, Steve Bocciarelli D (1967). An electron microscope study on primary periosteal bone. J Ultrastruct Res 18:605.

Ascenzi A, Francois C, Steve Bocciarelli D (1963). On the bone induced by estrogens in birds. J Ultrastruct Res 8:491.

Bachra BN (1967). Some colecular aspects of tissue calcification. Clin Orthop 51:199.

Bachra BN (1970). Calcification in vitro of collagenous model systems: chemical and electronmicroscopic aspects. Calcif Tiss Res 4 (suppl.):31.

Bernard GW (1972). Ultrastructural observations on initial calcification in dentine and enamel. J Ultrastruct Res 41:1.

Bernard GW, Pease DC (1969). An electron microscopic study of initial intramembranous osteogenesis. Am J Anat 125:271.

Bonucci E: Fine structure of early cartilage calcification. J Ultrastruct Res 20:33.

Bonucci E (1969). Further investigation on the organic/inorganic relationships in calcifying cartilage. Calcif Tiss Res 3:38.

Bonucci E (1970). Fine structure and histochemistry of "calcifying globules" in epiphyseal cartilage. Z Zellforsch 103:192.

Bonucci E (1971). The locus of initial calcification in cartilage and bone. Clin Orthop 78:108.

Bonucci E (1975). The organic-inorganic relationships in calcified organic matrices. In "Physico-chemie et cristallographie des apatites d'intérêt biologique", Colloque n. 230 du CNRS, Paris p 231.

Bonucci E, De Matteis A (1968). Ultrastruttura della cartilagine epifisaria nello scorbuto sperimentale. II. La matrice organica ed il processo di calcificazione. Ortop Traumat Appar Motore 36:293.

Bonucci E, De Santis E (1980). Ultrastructure of osteoblastoma, with particular reference to calcification and matrix vesicles. In "Bone and tumors", Editions Médecine et Hygiène, Genève, p 232.

Bonucci E, Frollà G, Piacentini M, Piantoni L (1978). Presenza di materiale sudanofilo nella matrice ossea e cartilaginea e processo di calcificazione: indagini istochimiche ed ultrastrutturali. Riv Istochim Norm Pat 22:77.

Bonucci E, Gherardi G (1975). Histochemical and electron microscope investigations on medullary bone. Cell Tiss Res 163:81.

Bonucci E, Sadun R. An electron microscope study on experimental calcification of skeletal muscle. Clin Orthop 88:197.

Bonucci E, Sadun R (1973). Experimental calcification of the myocardium. Am J Pathol 71:167.

Bonucci E, Sadun R (1975). Dihydrotachysterol-induced aortic calcification. Clin Orthop 107:283.

Boskey AL (1978). The role of calcium-phospholipid-phosphate complexes in tissue mineralization. Metab Bone Dis Rel Res 1:137.

Boskey AL, Posner AS (1976). Extraction of a calcium-phospholipid-phosphate complex from bone. Calcif Tiss Res 19:273.

Boskey AL, Posner AS, Lane JM, Goldberg MR, Cordella DM (1980). Distribution of lipid associated with mineralization in the bovine epiphyseal growth plate. Arch Biochem Biophys 199:305.

Bowness JM (1968). Present concepts of the role of ground substance in calcification. Clin Orthop 59:233.

Brighton CT, Hunt RM (1978). Electron microscopic pyro-antimonate studies of matrix vesicles and mitochondria in the rachitic growth plate. Metab Bone Dis Rel Res 1:199.

Cameron DA (1963). The fine structure of bone and calcified cartilage. Clin Orthop 26:199.

Campo RD (1970). Protein-polysaccharides of cartilage and bone in health and disease. Clin Orthop 68:182.

Cooper RR, Milgram JW, Robinson RA (1966). Morphology of the osteon. An electron microscopic study. J Bone Joint Surg 48A:1239.

De Bernard B, Stagni N, Colautti I, Vittur F, Bonucci E (1977). Glycosaminoglycans and endochondral calcification. Clin Orthop 126:285.

Decker JD: An electron microscopic investigation of osteo-genesis in the embryonic chick. Am J Anat 118:591.

Deyl Z, Macek K, Vancikova O, Adam M (1979). The presence of γ-carboxyglutamic acid-containing protein in atheromatous aortae. Biochim Biophys Acta 581:307.

Dimuzio MT, Veis A (1978). Phosphorins-Mayor noncollagenous proteins of rat incisor dentine. Calcif Tiss Res 25:169.

Dudley HR, Spiro D (1961). The fine structure of bone cells. J Biophys Biochem Cytol 11:627.

Eisenmann DR, Glick PL (1972). Ultrastructure of initial crystal formation in dentine. J Ultrastruct Res 41:18.

Fitton Jackson S (1957). The fine structure of developing bone in the embryonic fowl. Proc Roy Soc B 146:270.

Glimcher MJ (1959). Molecular biology of mineralized tissues with particular reference to bone. Rev Mod Phys 31:359.

Glimcher MJ, Brickley-Parsons D, Kossiva D (1979). Phospho-peptides and γ-carboxyglutamic acid-containing peptides in calcified turkey tendon: Their absence in uncalcified tendon. Calcif Tiss Int 27:281.

Glimcher MJ, Krane SM (1968). The organization and structure of bone, and the mechanism of calcification. In Ramachandran SN (ed): "Treatise on collagen", Vol. 2B: Biology of collagen, Academic Press, London, p 67.

Hauschka PV, Lian JB, Gallop PM (1975). Direct identification of the calcium-binding amino acid, γ-carboxyglutamate, in mineralized tissue. Proc Nat Acad Sci 72:3925.

Höhling HJ (1969). Collagen mineralization in bone, dentine, cementum, and cartilage. Naturwissenschaft 56:466.

Irving JT (1969). The sudanophil material in the early stages of calcification. Archs Oral Biol 8:735.

Irving JT (1973). Theories of mineralization of bone. Clin Orthop 97:225.

Irving JT, Wuthier RE (1968). Histochemistry and biochemistry of calcification with special reference to the role of lipids. Clin Orthop 56:237.

Lehninger AL (1970). Mitochondria and calcium ion transport. Biochem J 119:129.

Levy RJ, Lian JB, Gallop P (1979). Atherocalcin, a γ-carboxyglutamic acid containing protein from atherosclerotic plaque. Biochem Biophys Res Comm 91:41.

Lian JB, Skinner M, Glimcher MJ, Gallop P (1976). The presence of γ-carboxyglutamic acid in the proteins associated with ectopic calcification. Biochem Biophys Res Conn 73:349.

Robinson RA, Cameron DA (1956). Electron microscopy of cartilage and bone matrix at the distal epiphyseal line of the femur in the newborn infant. J Biophys Biochem Cytol 2 (suppl.): 253.

Sayegh FS, Davis RW, Solomon GC (1974). Mitochondrial role in cellular mineralization. J Dent Res 53:581.

Schiffmann E, Martin GR, Miller EJ (1968). Matrices that calcify. In Schraer H (ed): "Biological calcification", Appleton-Century-Crofts, New York, p 27.

Schubert M, Pras M (1968). Ground substance proteinpolysaccharides and precipitation of calcium phosphate. Clin Orthop 60:235.

Shapiro IM (1970). The phospholipids of mineralized tissues. I. Mammalian compact bone. Calcif Tiss Res 5:21.

Shuttleworth A, Veis A (1972). The isolation of anionic phosphoproteins from bovine cortical bone via the periodate solubilization of bone collagen. Biochim Biophys Acta 257:414.

Slavkin HC, Croissant R, Bringas P (1972). Epithelial-mesenchymal interactions during odontogenesis. III. A simple method for the isolation of matrix vesicles. J Cell Biol 53:841.

Sobel AE (1955). Local factors in the mechanism of calcification. Ann N Y Acad Sci 60:713.

Stagni N, Furian G, Vittur F, Zanetti M, De Bernard B (1979). Enzymatic properties of the Ca^{2+}-binding glycoprotein isolated from preosseous cartilage. Calcif Tiss Int 29:27.

Urist MR (1964). Recent advances in physiology of calcification. J Bone Joint Surg 46A:889.

Urist MR (1966). Origins of current ideas about calcification. Clin Orthop 44:13.

Veis A, Spector AR, Zamoscianyk H (1972). The isolation of an EDTA-soluble phosphoprotein from mineralizing bovine dentin. Biochim Biophys Acta 257:404.

Vittur F, De Bernard B (1973). Alkaline phosphatase activity associated to a calcium binding glycoprotein from calf scapula cartilage. FEBS Lett 38:87.

Vittur F, Pugliarello MC, De Bernard B (1972). The calcium binding properties of a glycoprotein isolated from preosseous cartilage. Biochem Biophys Res Comm 48:143.

Vogel JJ, Boyan-Salyers BD (1976). Acidic lipids associated with the local mechanism of calcification. Clin Orthop 118:230.

Weidmann SM (1963). Calcification of skeletal tissues. Int Rev Connect Tiss Res 1:339.

Wuthier RE (1968). Lipids of mineralizing epiphyseal tissues in the bovine fetus. J Lipid Res 9:68.

Wuthier RE (1969). A zonal analysis of inorganic and organic constituents of the epiphysis during endochondral calcification. Calcif Tiss Res 4:20.

Connective Tissue Research:
Chemistry, Biology, and Physiology, Pages 125–129
© **1981 Alan R. Liss, Inc., 150 Fifth Avenue, New York, N.Y. 10011**

TISSUE SPECIFIC DIFFERENCES OF COLLAGEN

Jürgen Rauterberg

Institut für Arterioskleroseforschung an der
Universität
Westring 3, 44 Münster, GFR

It is one of the characteristics of connective tissue
that in spite of very different functions and different
properties and morphologic features there is a relatively
high degree of conformity among the components of the extracellular matrix. The main proteins in most connective tissues
are: collagen, proteoglycans, certain glycoproteins and
elastin

The functional versatility is rendered possible by the
fact that each of the components in itself has a high potential to vary in structure and function, and collagen is
probably the best known example how proteins can achieve
functional versatility in different ways. In case of this
protein the possibilities of structural variations can be
summarised into three groups:

(1) Heterogeneity is due to the existence of several
    genetically different "collagen types; their occur-
    rence and quantitative ratio varies in different
    connective tissues

(2) Biosynthesis of collagen does involve a number of
    - partly enzymatically controlled - post-translati-
    onal modifications; by changing enzyme activity or
    specifity a certain degree of variability is
    possible

(3) Collagen is involved into various interactions with
    other components of the extracellular matrix. Pro-
    perties of collagen are greatly influenced by those
    interactions, especially the formation of fibrils
    is very sensitive to the presence of other compo-
    nents as it is known from various in vitro experi-
    ments

Certainly the most obvious tissue-specific differences are
caused by the occurrence of collagen molecules built up by
different polypeptide chains with distinct amino acid sequences. But none of these different collagen types is restricted
to only one organ or one kind of connective tissue; various
tissues contain the same collagen types; only their quantitative ratio and - in certain limits - there morphologic
appearance may be different.

Only few and according to their function rather specialized tissues confine themselves to one type of collagen.
Bone and tendon, for instance, have practically only type I
in their extracellular matrix. Type II collagen was believed
for long time to represent the only collagen in hyaline
cartilage; recently, however, the occurrence of two further
collagenous polypeptides was shown (Burgeson and Hollister,
1979)

The major part of connective tissues contains several
types of collagen within the same areas of their extracellular matrix. Type III collagen is always occurring together
with type I. It is known from in vitro experiments to form
fibrils wich are nearly identical to type I derived fibrils
(Wiedemann et.al., 1975); there have been numerous discussions
which morphologic structure of extracellular matrices may
represent type III collagen. Suggestions that the network
of reticular fibrils in parenchymal organs as liver or spleen
is formed only by type III could not be confirmed by immun-
histology, which indicates occurrence of types I and III in
these areas. Recent findings in our laboratory suggest that
at least in some tissues type I and III may form composite
fibrils: From vessel walls and from uterus leiomyomata cross-
link-containing peptides were isolated which link α1(I) and
1(III) (Henkel and Glanville, 1980).

Type IV and V are currently referred to as basement membrane
collagens, Basement membrane is primarily defined as a morphologic term. Tissue-specific differences, e.g. between
glomerular and smooth muscle cell basement membranes, are
known from electronmicroscopy. Whereas type IV is known to
be the main collagenous component in a number of basement
membranes, the occurrence and role of type V is still unclear.
Recently polypeptide chains of type IV have been isolated
from several tissues; typical tissue-specific differences
cannot be deduced from these results (Dixit, 1978; Kresina
and Miller, 1979; Sage and others, 1979; Dixit, 1980)
Type V derived αA and αB chains isolated from amniotic membranes and aorta do not show tissue-specific differences

according to their amino acid composition, their cyanogen bromide pattern and the cross-striation patterns of long spacing crystalltes. On the other hand, differences in the ratio of αA and αB have been reported (Rhodes and Miller, 1978) and a third Type V-associated chain seems to be restricted to certain tissues (Sage and Bornstein, 1979).

As we have seen, a great deal of tissue-specific differences are due to the occurence of geneticaly distinct collagen molecules. Due to the fascinating results which have been obtained on this topic another aspect of tissue-specific heterogeneity has been put back a little during the last years: a heterogeneity which is caused by differences in post-translational modification during the biosynthesis of collagen molecules. Several important structural features are introduced by enzymatically controlled intra- and extracellular processing and the activity as well as - to a less extent - also the specifity of involved enzymes represents an important factor in the regulation of properties of collagen. Table 1 summarizes the post-translational steps of collagen biosynthesis; in the last column their possible relevance for tissue-specific heterogeneity is mentioned.

Step	Enzyme involved	Biological Significance	Tissue specific differences
Removal of hydrophobic N-terminal "Pre"-peptide	ER-Membrane bound Protease	Transport through membrane of ER	—
Hydroxylation of proline	Prolylhydroxylases	Stability of tripelhelix Tripelhelix formation at 37C	Degree of hydroxylation skin bone, tendon
Hydroxylation of Lysine	Lysylhydroxylase	Stability of crosslinks Essential for glycosylation	Degree of Hydroxylation bone tendon skin
Glycosylation of hydroxylysine	Galactosyltransferase, Glycosyltransferase	Stability of crosslinks (?), Interaction with matrix components (?) Regulation of fibrilformation (?)	Degree of Glycosylation and localization of carbohydrates
Assembly; disulfide bonding Tripelhelixformation	—	Essential for secretion Stops hydroxylation and glycosylation	—
Cleavage of procollagen peptides Fibril formation	Procollagenpeptidases	Essential for fibre formation	Thickness, length and shape of fibrils and fibres
Aldehyde formation Crosslinking	Lysyloxidase —	Essential for crosslink formation Strengh and stability of fibrils	Degree of crosslinking and chemistry and localization of crosslinks

Table 1. Post-translational steps of collagen biosynthesis

The majority of differences are poorly understood in their functional meaning. A lower degree of hydroxylation of proline in skin, as compared to aorta and bone (Rauterberg, unpublished results) may be simply due to different tissue temperatures, without any function. Differences in the hydroxylation of lysine, however, are very important for the stability of intermolecular crosslinks because crosslinks derived from two hydroxylysine residues are more stable than those from two lysine or one lysine and hydroxylysine. In fact, a higher degree of lysine hydroxylation has been found for bone collagen and to a less extent also for tendon collagen as compared to skin type I (Stoltz et al., 1973) Not only the degree of hydroxylation, but also the localisation of OH-groups is of great importance: As the terminal non-helical regions are preferably involved in crosslinking, hydroxylation of lysine in this region as it has found in bone collagen does certainly contribute to crosslink stability. Specific localization of hydroxylysine in the region of $\alpha 1(I)CB3$ has been described for cornea collagen (Panjwani and Harding, 1978)

The functional meaning of glycosylation is still poorly understood, it may be important for fibril formation ; highly glycosylated collagens do form thin fibrils (Spiro, 1969) – and for crosslink stability - some of the crosslink compounds have found to be glycosylated.

Intermolecular crosslinking reveals a high degree of tissue specific heterogeneity, as well as the number and the chemical nature is concerned. Various tissues have been shown to possess a specific pattern of crosslink compounds and it would be beyond the scope of this introduction to discuss differences in degree of chemical nature or the localization of intermolecular crosslinks. It should be pointed, however, to the fact that regulation of crosslink formation happens to a great deal by intracellular modifications of procollagen; on the other hand, extracellular steps are also important e.g. the activity of lysyloxidase which again may be influenced by several factors.

Extracellular factors probably play a very important role in the regulation of fibril formation. This process is far from being understood, though great progress has been made in understanding principles of fibril structure. Certainly various extracellular factors do influence thickness, shape and density of fibrils and it is still a mystery how nature achieves the regular packing of fibrils and their equal diameter in certain tissues. Interactions between collagen and other components, including cell membranes, probably cause a great deal of tissue-specific differences; These interactions certainly will be a very important topic of research in the future.

Burgeson RE, Hollister DW (1979). Collagen heterogeneity in human cartilage: identification of several new collagen chains. Biochem Biophys Res Comm 87:1124.

Dixit SN (1978). Isolation and characterization of two collagenous components from anterior lens capsule. FEBS-Letters 85:153.

Dixit SN (1980). Type IV collagens. Isolation and characterization of two structurally distinct collagenous chains from bovine kidney cortices. Europ J Biochem 106:563.

Henkel W, Glanville R (1980). Covalent crosslinking between molecules of type I and type III collagen. The involvement of the N-terminal non-helical regions of the α1(I) and α1(III) chains in formation of intermicrofibrillar crosslinks. Europ J Biochem subm.

Kresina TF, Miller EJ (1979). Isolation and characterization of basement membrane collagen from human placenta. Tissue evidence for the presence of two genetically distinct collagen chains. Biochemistry 18:3089.

Panjwani A, Harding JJ (1978). Chymotryptic and tryptic peptides of fragment α1-CB 3 from bovine corneal collagen. Pinpointing the sites of hexose attachment. Biochem J 171:697.

Rhodes RK, Miller EJ (1978). Physi hemical characterization and molecular organization of the collagen A and B chains. Biochemistry 17:3442.

Sage H, Bornstein P (1979). Characterization of a novel collagen chain in human placenta and its relation to AB - collagen. Biochemistry 18:3815.

Sage H, Woodbury RG, Bornstein P(1979). Structural studies on human type IV collagen. J Biochem 254:9893.

Spiro RG (1969). Characterization and quantitative determination of the hydroxylysine-linked carbohydrate units of several collagens. J Biol Chem 244:6o2.

Stoltz M, Furthmayr H, Timpl R (1973). Increased lysine hydroxylation in rat bone and tendon collagen and localization the additional residues. Biochim Biophys Acta 310:461.

Wiedemann H, Chung E, Fujii T, Miller EJ, Kühn K (1975). Comparative electron-microscopic studies on type-III and type-I collagens. Europ J Biochem 51:363.

Connective Tissue Research:
Chemistry, Biology, and Physiology, Pages 131–133
© 1981 Alan R. Liss, Inc., 150 Fifth Avenue, New York, N.Y. 10011

CHEMICAL AND IMMUNOHISTOLOGIC CHARACTERIZATION OF COLLAGENOUS
COMPONENTS IN THE NORMAL AND DISEASED SKIN

Lutz Weber

Department of Dermatology, University of Ulm,
79 Ulm, FRG

The skin has, on the light microscopic level, a characteristic anatomical stratification. It can be sub-divided into the
epidermis, which consists of epithelial cells, and the dermis, which consists mainly of connective tissue and includes
the major part of the skin. Immediately beneath the epidermis
is the epidermal basement membrane, which is part of the
epidermo-dermal junction. The dermis comprises two compart-
ments, the papillary and the reticular layer. The papillary
layer is a small zone of connective tissue underlying the
epidermal basement membrane. It shows a loose meshwork of
thin collagen fibrils. By contrast the reticular layer contains coarse collagen bundles and comprises the major part of
the dermis. Finally there is the subcutaneous fat layer, which
is separated from the dermis by the dermo-subcutaneous interface.

The human dermis consists by over 70% of connective tissue. But apart from this there are other important functional
structures, for example the adnexa, such as hair follicles
with the musculus errector pili, sebaceous glands adjoining
to the hair follicle, eccrine sweat glands above the dermo-
subcutaneous interface, and of course blood vessels, lympha-
tics and nerve fibres. Thus the skin is actually an organ
with a variety of distinct functions. It has accordingly a
highly organized structure, which is closely related to a
specific distribution of its connective tissue components.
Investigation of these components may help to understand the
different functions of the skin and contribute to establish
the role of the different collagen types.

Apart from type II collagen, all the collagen types iden-

tified as yet in the human organism are present in the skin.
The major interstitial collagens in the skin are type I and
III collagen. They are present in about equal amounts in fetal skin, whereas the proportion of type III collagen in the
adult skin is about 15%(Epstein 1974). Types I and III collagen and type III procollagen are distributed all over the
dermis and the subcutaneous fat tissue. By contrast type I
procollagen stains in immunohistologic studies in a linear
fashion beneath the epidermis and around other structures derived from the epithelium, such as hair follicles. The reason
for this selective staining behaviour is at present unclear.
It has been assumed from immunohistologic studies that type
III collagen predominates in the papillary layer (Meigel et
al. 1977), but this finding could not as yet be confirmed by
biochemical data. The human skin contains also about 5%
α1(I)-trimer (Uitto 1979). This percentage is even higher
in fetal skin. At present there are however no data with respect to the histotopic distribution of this molecular form.

As for skin diseases, there are apparently no significant changes in the relative proportion of type I versus type
III collagen in most pathologic conditions investigated as
yet. An altered type I/III ratio has however been found in
early stages of fibrotic and neoplastic processes and in hereditary diseases. The relative proportion of type III collagen is increased in early scar formation and in fibrotic tumors, such as fibrosarcoma. An obvious reduction in type III
collagen and procollagen was reported in Ehlers-Danlos syndrome type IV (Pope et al. 1975). Extensive studies have been
carried out on systemic sclerosis. In this disease collagen
production is conspicuously increased in fibroblasts derived
from the dermo-subcutaneous interface. However no alteration
in the proportion of type I versus type III collagen could be
ascertained by biochemical means (Krieg et al. 1980).

Soon after its characterization in fetal membranes, AB
or type V collagen was identified in human skin as well
(Chung et al. 1976). Furthermore it could be shown that type
V collagen is present in the three layers of the skin, i.e.
the papillary layer, the reticular layer and the subcutaneous
fat layer, and that fibroblasts derived from each of these
three layers are able to produce α A and α B chains (Weber et
al. 1980)

The more recently characterized basement membrane (b.m.)
proteins, type IV collagen(Timpl et al. 1978) and laminin
(Timpl et al. 1979), could be localized by immunohistology
in a variety of basement membranes in the skin. These two

components line in strict co-distribution whole tissue complexes such as the epidermis, the hair follicles and sebaceous gland lobes and also surround single cells such as smooth muscle cells, adipocytes and Schwann cells. As for skin diseases it could be shown that in basal cell carcinoma, a malignant infiltrating tumor of the skin, the tumor cell formations are surrounded by an almost continuous b.m. containing both type IV collagen and laminin. This is of interest with regard to the fact that this tumor almost never gives rise to metastasis. In bullous pemphigoid, a common blistering disease in elderly people, type IV collagen (which is a constituent of the lamina densa of the epidermal b.m.) and laminin (which is a constituent of the lamina lucida of the epidermal b.m.) could be located on the ground of the blister, which is an important information for the localization of the pathogenetic focus in this disease.

Chung E, Rhodes RK, Miller EJ (1976). Isolation of three collagenous components of probable basement membrane origin from several tissues. Biochem Biophys Res Commun 71:1167

Epstein EH Jr (1974). $[\alpha 1(III)]_3$ human skin collagen. Release by pepsin digestion and preponderance in fetal life. J Biol Chem 249:3225

Krieg T, Luderschmidt C, Weber L, Müller PK, Braun-Falco O (1980). Scleroderma fibroblasts: some aspects of in vitro assessment of collagen synthesis. Arch Derm Res. In press.

Meigel WN, Gay S, Weber L (1977). Dermal architecture and collagen type distribution. Arch Derm Res 259:1

Pope FM, Martin GR, Lichtenstein JR, Penttinen R, Gerson B, Rowe DW, McKusick VA (1975). Patients with Ehlers-Danlos syndrome type IV lack type III collagen. Proc Natl Acad Sci USA 72:1314

Timpl R, Martin GR, Bruckner P, Wick G, Wiedemann H (1978). Nature of the collagenous protein in a tumor basement membrane. Eur J Biochem 84:43

Timpl R, Rohde H, Gehron Robey P, Rennard SJ, Foidart JM, Martin GR (1979). Laminin - a glycoprotein from basement membranes. J Biol Chem 254:9933

Uitto J (1979). Collagen polymorphism: isolation and partial characterization of $\alpha 1(I)$-trimer molecules in normal human skin. Arch Biochem Biophys 192:371

Weber L, Kirsch E, Krieg T, Wiestner M, Müller PK (1980). Type V collagen in skin - characterization of the α-chains and study of synthesis. J Invest Derm 76,6:452

Connective Tissue Research:
Chemistry, Biology, and Physiology, Pages 135–138
© 1981 Alan R. Liss, Inc., 150 Fifth Avenue, New York, N.Y. 10011

STRUCTURE AND ORGANIZATION OF CONNECTIVE MATRIX IN THE
LIVER: CORRELATION BETWEEN MORPHOLOGICAL AND CHEMICAL DATA

S. PEYROL, J.A. GRIMAUD

Laboratoire de Pathologie Cellulaire du Foie –
C.N.R.S. – ERA 819 – INSTITUT PASTEUR
77, rue Pasteur, 69007 LYON , FRANCE.

In the liver, the connective tissue has two main functions : *support and mediation*

Support function : is assumed first by the *Glison's capsule* which overlaps the liver by a sheet of connective tissue, and then the *portal connective tree* : this latter sheathes together vascular afferences (portal and arterial) and biliary efferences (biliary tree) and precisely distributes them into the hepatic parenchyma in order to establish the acinar organization of the liver (RAPPAPORT A.M., 1958).

Mediation : between blood and hepatocytes passes through *space of Disse*, this thin connective layer, associated to the endothelial sinusoidal wall and bathing the vascular pole of the hepatocytes : this connective unit is the key of trophic and regulative blood-hepatocytes exchanges and one essential site for immunological events.

Glisson's capsule, portal tree and Disse space form a continuous network which answers "en bloc" to any liver damage (dysfunctional, toxic, viral or parasitic) by modification both of its connective cell components and of its connective matrix.

Today, three main methods are used to characterize the molecular components of the human liver connective matrix : - biochemical studies
- ultrastructural morphological studies
- tissular immunolabelling

Biochemical studies : have now established the tissular specific composition and the quantitative estimation of the
main collagenous proteins of the human liver (ROJKIND M et
al., 1979; CHEVALIER O. and col., 1978).

In normal human liver, interstitial collagens are represented by TYPE I and TYPE III ; basement membrane collagens are
represented by TYPE IV, TYPE V (AB) and TYPE E which resem-
ble respectively to basement collagens extracted from human placenta and skin, and from human aorta. In cirrhotic
liver, an additional collagen was identified as a trimer
of α1 TYPE I collagen.

Normal liver contains rather equal amounts of TYPE I, III
and basement membrane collagens and the ratio TYPE I/
TYPE III suggests a slight predominance of TYPE III. In
cirrhotic liver, all collagen types are increased and their
relative ratio is only modified in severe cirrhosis :
TYPE I/TYPE III ratio suggests predominance of TYPE I.

Ultrastructural morphological studies : give visualization
of the macromolecular systems and show their interrelation
and mode of organization in situ :

The fibrous form of collagen with its characteristic 640 $\overset{\circ}{A}$
periodicity is well known. In normal liver, fibers appear
either isolated in Disse space, or grouped in bundles in
Glisson's capsule and portal spaces.
The fibrillar form of collagen is also well represented
first in portal spaces, among connective matrix and in association with vascular and biliary tracts, and then in Disse
space between endothelial cell wall and vascular pole of
hepatocytes.
The basement membrane form of collagen is present only in
portal spaces around vascular bed along endothelial (portal venous and arterial) and epithelial biliary cells.
In the cirrhotic process, fibrosis develops everywhere :
in Glisson's capsule and portal spaces mainly, large dense
bundles of fibrous collagen extend and form fibrous septa
which penetrate into the lobule leading to the nodular
architecture of the liver, that is *DENSE CONNECTIVE MATRIX
ORGANIZATION* . In portal spaces, rather around vascular
and biliary tracts, and in Disse's space, fibrillar and
basement membrane like collagens form a loose reticular
connective network, that is the *LOOSE CONNECTIVE MATRIX
ORGANIZATION* (GRIMAUD J.A. and col., 1977). An unusual
form of collagen (hyperfibre) is inconstantly present in
fibrotic livers (PEYROL S. and col., 1976) whose pathologi-

cal significance is still unknown.

Tissular immunolabelling allows to correlate biochemical and morphological findings. Ultrastructural immunoperoxidase allows to determine the molecular nature of the macromolecular systems and immunofluorescence reveals the histological localization of each collagen type (GAY S. and col., 1975 ; KENT G. and col., 1976 ; RAUTERBERG J. and col., 1978 ; GRIMAUD J.A. and col., 1980).

TYPE I corresponds to the fibrous form of collagen and is present in portal space mainly and to a less extent in Disse space, as bundles of fibers. In cirrhotic livers, TYPE I deposit is enhanced and is the essential component of dense connective matrix organization.

TYPE III corresponds to the fibrillar form of collagen which develops as a reticular network around vascular and biliary tracts in portal space and around sinusoidal wall in Disse space. In cirrhotic process, TYPE III deposit is enhanced and is the essential component of loose connective matrix organization. Type B collagen has the same location as TYPES I and III and follows their quantitative changes in fibrotic process (BIEMPICA L. and col., 1980).

TYPE IV and fibronectin correspond mainly to the laminar form of collagen present in portal space along limiting, vascular, biliary and hepatocytic cell plates and, to a less extent, to the basement membrane like material scattered in the connective matrix ; they are also present in Disse space in close association with the endothelial cells. In cirrhotic liver, enhancement of TYPE IV deposit is especially important in Disse space and in portal connective matrix where it contributes to the loose connective matrix organization. The distinctive characters of LAMININ are its absence in Disse space and its close association to portal and septal limiting hepatocytic cell plate (HAHN E. and col., 1979).

The biochemical evidence of the different types of collagen has transformed our knowledge on connective tissue and tissular fibrosis. Now, it appears that, more than quantity, the notion of quality of fibrosis is important to appreciate its evolutive potential or its stability : predominance of TYPE I in DCMO can be related to the stability of such deposits since predominance of TYPE III and TYPE IV in LCMO traduces its evolutive and remodelling characters.

The fibrotic process might be now appreciated in terms of evolutive prognosis and susceptibility to therapeutic agents. Different directions of research might now give significative progress in tissular fibrosis knowledge :
- regulative mechanisms of fibrogenesis ;
- seric markers of fibrosis destabilisation ;
- cellular control of fibrolysis ;
- mechanism of action of anti-fibrotic molecules.

Biempica L, Morecki R, Wu CH and col (1980). Am J Pathol 98 : 592.

Chevalier O, Herbage D, Grimaud JA (1978). 6th colloquium of the Federation of European Connective Tissue Clubs 1 Créteil CNRS ed 82.

Gay S, Fietzek PP, Remberger K and col (1975). Klin Wochens-schr 53 : 205.

Grimaud JA, Borojevic R, Peyrol S (1977). Biol Cell 29 : 24a

Hahn E, Wick G, Pencv D and Timpl R (1980). Gut 21 : 63.

Kent G, Gay S, Inouye T and col (1976). Proc Nat Acad Sci USA 73 : 3719.

Peyrol S, Grimaud JA and Borojevic R (1976). C R Acad Sci PARIS 282 : 333.

Rauterberg J, Voss B, Pott G (1978). 6th Colloquium of the Federation of European Connective Tissue Clubs 1 Créteil CNRS et 125.

Rappaport AM (1958). Anat Rec 130 : 673.

Rojkind M and col (1979). Gastroenterol 76 : 710.

Grimaud JA, Druguet M, Peyrol S and col (1980). J Histochem Cytochem in press.

Connective Tissue Research:
Chemistry, Biology, and Physiology, Pages 139–140
© 1981 Alan R. Liss, Inc., 150 Fifth Avenue, New York, N.Y. 10011

CONNECTIVE TISSUE COMPONENTS OF THE EYE

Otto Schmut

Univ.-Augenklinik, Auenbruggerplatz 4,
A-8036 Graz, Austria.

The different transparent tissues of the eye have been extensively investigated in the last years and a short review on the many studies should be presented here.

CORNEA

Collagen type I, type IV and A and B chains have been clearly proven in cornea. The content of type II and especially type III collagen is a point of controversy in many papers. However, type III collagen gained importance in the pathology of the cornea. Sections of keratoconus corneas showed in immunofluorescence type III collagen in a greater quantity than normal corneas. In contrast, in tissue cultures fibroblasts of both normal and keratoconus corneas synthesize 5-10% of collagen type III and there was no difference in the products synthesized by normal and keratoconus fibroblasts.

The differences seem to be dependent on that cultures of corneal fibroblasts synthesize collagen types in a different proportion than intact corneas. The culture conditions under which the corneal fibroblasts synthesize type III collagen are the same under which they lose the ability to synthesize the corneal type keratan sulfate. Therefore, in tissue culture corneal cells do not produce the glycosaminoglycan distribution pattern as expected from the analysis of corneal tissue.

VITREOUS BODY

Pepsin-solubilized vitreous body collagen can be separated by differential salt precipitation into different hydroxyproline containing components with different polyacrylamidegel-electrophoretic patterns and different CNBr-derived peptides. Therefore, we suggest that bovine vitreous body collagen consists of a mixture of different collagen types.

Hyaluronic acid of bovine vitreous body can be purified by a non-enzymic method using cold 5% trichloroacetic acid to remove the bulk of proteins and further purification with activated CH-Sepharose 4B. With this method we obtained a highly purified hyaluronic acid and we could demonstrate by immunochemical methods that the remaining protein represents a hyaluronic acid specific protein.

LENS CAPSULE

In the last few years it has been established that lens capsule collagen represents a family of collagens and until now different α-chains have been isolated from lens capsules. A classification of lens capsule collagens will surely be done in the future.

Connective Tissue Research:
Chemistry, Biology, and Physiology, Pages 141–149
© 1981 Alan R. Liss, Inc., 150 Fifth Avenue, New York, N.Y. 10011

THE EVOLUTION OF CONNECTIVE TISSUE. PHYLOGENETIC DISTRIBUTION
AND MODIFICATIONS DURING DEVELOPMENT

Robert GARRONE

Laboratoire d'Histologie et Biologie Tissulaire
(L.A. C.N.R.S. 244), Université Claude Bernard,
43, Bd. 11 novembre, 69622 VILLEURBANNE Cedex,
FRANCE

The connective tissue of higher vertebrates is very well
defined at the molecular level. The collagen types, the
proteoglycan structures, the elastic fibres and the different
glycoproteins have all been identified and characterized. The
situation is, however, very different in invertebrates as
there is very little available information. Only very few
studies give biochemical and morphological data at the same
time. The lack of knowledge in this domain is surprising, as
95% of all animal species are invertebrates, however it
limits the present review.

During animal evolution, connective tissue has appeared
simultaneously with organized multicellular life, that is
with the first metazoa (Garrone, 1978). At first, it was not
the same as it is now in higher animals, even if the most
important molecules, collagen and glycoproteins have changed
only very little (Adams, 1978; Bairati, 1972; Mathews, 1975).
Each zoological group has its own variations, but nevertheless
there are constant factors which are all invaluable keys to
understanding connective tissue, its structure in adults as
well as its development in embryos.

Most comparative studies of connective tissue have
considered collagen above all. The interest is legitimate as
collagen is the major protein in the tissue, but this only
shows part of the story. For a wider view, the evolution of
connective tissue can be considered at three levels: the
macromolecular structures developing in the organism; then
the intercellular matrices; and finally the limits of these
matrices, i.e. the membranes and cell surfaces, sites of

.

cell-matrix interactions.

CONNECTIVE TISSUE SYSTEMS IN THE SCALE OF THE ORGANISM

The grouping of certain macromolecules and their eventual association with mineral compounds results in macroscopic structures stretching throughout the organism. All types of connective tissue molecules can be involved in these structures: collagen, whether or not mineralized (skeletons, cuticles...); proteoglycans (cartilage...); structural glycoproteins and elastin (elastic laminae and fibres...).

Almost each invertebrate group has its own specific collagen organized in macroscopic structures. These may be, for example, spongin fibres in sponges or the internal skeletal rods of cnidarians, with skeletal functions; the cuticles of worms, for protection; the byssus of some molluscs, for fixation. Very little is known about these collagens. A few studies on the cuticles of *Ascaris* (Evans *et al.*, 1976) and *Nereis* (Kimura and Tanzer, 1977) suggest in these collagens the existence of particular polypeptide chains. The molecular weight for each chain seems to be very high in *Nereis* (470,000), lower in *Ascaris* (52,000) where each chain would also contain non-collagenous domains, many disulfide bonds and might be bent and twisted into a triple helix. These collagens have no equivalent in vertebrates, except perhaps in the most primitive of them, fish. Fish, indeed, have elastoïdin rods and some more primitive groups (i.e. dogfish) have collagenous cases around their eggs.

On the other hand, in vertebrates, the mineralized collagens are most developed in teeth and bones. Unlike the first described structures, these mineralized collagens do not seem to exist in invertebrates. In a few cases (cnidarians, echinoderms...), the collagen fibres are found in calcified structures (containing calcium carbonate) but these are simply surrounded by the mineral and not impregnated with it. This was demonstrated in cnidarians (Ledger and Franc, 1978) and it may be the case in echinoderms too (Pucci-Minafra *et al.*, 1978). Even if bone is characteristic of vertebrates, its embryonic precursor, cartilage, is found in some invertebrates such as annelids and molluscs (Person and Philpott, 1969). In spite of the wide distribution of collagen and glycosamino-glycans in invertebrates (Hunt, 1970; Mathews, 1975) it is surprising to find that the formation of cartilage is not common.

In vertebrates, elastin and structural glycoproteins
form an interconnected system: the elastic system fibres.
It is composed of elastic, elaunin and oxytalan fibres
(Cotta-Pereira et al., 1978). This system gives (among other
things) elasticity to the skin and assures correct functioning of blood vessels. Elastin itself has not been found in
invertebrates (Sage and Gray, 1977), but pre-elastic fibres
can be detected. These fibres, of the oxytalan and perhaps
elaunin type can be shown by certain elastic fibre stains,
but only after oxidation (Elder, 1973) or tannic acid treatment
(Locke and Huie, 1975). Electron microscopy reveals above all
that the fibres are made up of bundles of microfibrils, thus
confirming their similarity with oxytalan fibres. The main
"elastic fibres" found in invertebrates would therefore be in
fact incomplete, or immature elastic fibres, characteristic
of elastogenesis in vertebrates. The organization of elastic
elements during evolution has probably depended on two major
events: living freely, requiring much movement; and the
appearance of a closed vascular system. Thus, in sponges, which
are sedentary animals, there are no elastic elements. In some
cnidarians living fixed, but changing considerably in volume,
the structural glycoproteins begin to form microfibrils, but
these stay dispersed (Franc, 1979). It is only in jellyfish
and ctenophores, which are pelagic animals, that the bundles
of microfibrils, characteristic of oxytalan fibres, can be found
(Elder, 1973). Other elastic systems, with no equivalent any-
where else, develop specifically in certain groups: the best
known is resilin in insects.

THE EVOLUTION OF INTERCELLULAR MATRICES

It is perhaps at this level that the most is known,
especially concerning collagen. In fact, even in sponges, the
intercellular matrices have all the essential constituants,
except for elastin (Garrone, 1978) and they vary only very
little even up to the vertebrates.

In view of present knowledge about collagen polymorphism,
one may wonder if one type of collagen may be more "primitive"
than another. In fact, in vertebrates, the first synthesis of
collagen corresponds to the deposit of a basement membrane in
the embryo (Low, 1967; Hay, 1973; Leivo et al., 1980). Type IV
collagen has indeed been detected in these embryonic structures

(Adamson and Ayers, 1979). This synthesis is rapidly followed
by the synthesis of type I and type III interstitial collagens
(Leivo *et al.*, 1980). Basement membrane collagens have been
compared to invertebrate collagens because of the similar
amino acid compositions, the presence of 3-hydroxyproline, of
cysteine, high contents of glycosylated hydroxylysine and,
sometimes, linkage with heteropolysaccharides. In fact, as
emphasized by Adams (1978), even if the comparison may be valid
for a particular invertebrate collagen, it cannot be generalized.
In other respects, if this comparison may be suggested by
biochemical studies, it is challenged by morphological observations establishing that invertebrates possess in general both
basement membranes and fibrillar collagens.

Collagen fibrils are present in nearly all invertebrate
species (Garrone, 1978). In the most primitive invertebrates
(sponges, coelenterates, flat worms...) the fibrils are less
organized than those of vertebrates. Their diameter is small
(20 nm) and their transverse banding is only faintly indicated.
A subperiod of 22 nm (that is about D/3) is often clearly marked
(Garrone, 1978) and could represent the expression of a primor-
dial collagen gene as suggested by Hofmann and his coworkers
(1980). With the annelids, the final morphology seems to be
acquired: the diameters are larger and the transverse banding
resembles that of vertebrate collagen fibrils. From the cnidarians onwards, and in the few cases where the molecular structure
has been analyzed, the molecules constantly seem to be formed of
three identical α_1 chains. These collagens were particularly
well studied in cnidarians (Nordwig *et al.*, 1973) and in insects
(Ashhurst and Bailey, 1980) where they were compared to the
type I trimer. Such collagen has been characterized in vertebrates (Mayne *et al.*, 1975), in the adult as well as the embryo
(Jimenez *et al.*, 1977). This relationship has again been
confirmed by histoimmunofluorescence showing strong cross-
reactions between collagens of invertebrates (cnidarians,
annelids, molluscs...) and anti bovine type I anti serum
(unpublished results). However, α_2 chains have been found
in echinoderms (Pucci-Minafra *et al.*, 1978), molluscs and
arthropods (Kimura and Matsuura, 1974), that is in more complex
invertebrates.

The appearance of type II collagen in vertebrates coincides
with the development of proteoglycan-rich matrices, mainly in
regions of chondrogenesis (Linsenmayer *et al.*, 1973; Von der
Mark *et al.*, 1976) but also in vitreous body and cornea of the
eye (Von der Mark *et al.*, 1977). Until now, such collagen has
never been found in invertebrate cartilage.

Basement membranes are only found in invertebrates with well-structured tissues. They are not found in sponges, which have only weakly joining epithelia and no marked muscle cells. They first appear in cnidarians (Garrone et al., 1979) where they are more obvious underlining contractile differentiation of epithelial cells. They are again clearly marked around true muscle cells of ctenophores (Hernandez-Nicaise and Amsellem, 1980). From then onwards they are constantly found throughout all the animal kingdom. In some groups, such as the rotifers they are probably the only collagenous structures (Clément, 1980). Biochemical analysis of insect collagens showed that, as well as fibrillar collagen, there is also one which resembles the vertebrate type IV (Ashhurst and Bailey, 1980). Even if basement membrane collagens are not the most primitive, their presence can still be related to stable cell differentiation. Finally, the existence of a basement membrane probably expresses the need for a definite microenvironment, essential to functions such as epithelial conduction and muscular contraction. In this rspect, it is interesting to notice that some vertebrate basement membrane collagens have been related to muscular differentiation (Von der Mark and Von der Mark, 1978; Bailey et al., 1979).

CELL-MATRIX INTERACTIONS

As soon as cells group together to form multicellular units cell interactions become essential for coordination. These interactions were found even before the formation of a structured intercellular matrix, for example in slime molds (Gerisch, 1979). These direct cell interactions are still found in all metazoa where they are involved in all morphogenetic phenomena. In sponges, these mechanisms have been studied in detail (Van de Vyvers, 1979). It is interesting to notice that, already at this level, these interactions depend on glycosylation (Müller et al., 1979), that is on reactions much used in the biosynthesis of the intercellular matrices. The specific recognition of the sugars involved may be due to membrane lectins (Monsigny et al., 1979) which are present in sponges. Some of the intramembrane particles seen after freeze-fracture of sponge cells, no doubt correspond to these molecules (Garrone and Lethias, 1980).

In addition to these direct cell-cell interactions, there are, in metazoa, indirect interactions via the intercellular matrices. Several studies have stressed the importance of these matrices for cell differentiation (Slavkin and Greulich, 1975; Reddi, 1976) and as active substratum promoting cell behavior (Hay, 1973). Recently, cell surface glycoproteins, the fibronectins, were described in vertebrates. They can act as intermediates between cells and the components of intercellular matrices (Vaheri et al., 1978). They are also of importance during embryogenesis (Critchley et al., 1979). Research for fibronectin-like substances in sponges has proved positive (Labat-Robert et al., 1979). It can therefore be said that substances for cell-matrix interactions developed at the same time as the intercellular matrix itself.

CONCLUSIONS

Through this evolution of connective tissue, one may first notice that collagen fibrils are well and truly fundamentally constant. The known exceptions are extremely rare. Fibrils existed before the basement membranes and acquired their final characteristics very early in evolution. Their original structure, based on molecules formed from three identical α chains, closely related to an α_1 type I trimer makes this collagen seem like an ancestral reminiscence rather than a curiosity. On the other hand, the different attempts of particular collagens to evolve were unsuccessful in that they vary from one group to another and they are no longer found in vertebrates.

The simultaneous appearance of basement membranes and stable tissue differentiation is a strong argument in favour of the idea that basement membrane collagens may have morphogenetic and functional influences.

In addition to the possibility of mineralizing collagen by calcium phosphate, another important of vertebrate connective tissue is the synthesis of elastin. This protein can then combine with the bundles of microfibrils, present even in almost the most primitive animals, to give the elastic system fibres.

Finally, right from the beginning, metazoa cells probably had all the membrane equipment needed for interactions with the intercellular matrices. Thus, the study of primitive animals shows that the evolution of connective tissue is a long story which has progressively been completed, starting initially in sponges from a well-defined plot.

REFERENCES

Adams E (1978). Invertebrate collagens. Science 202:591.

Adamson ED, Ayers SE (1979). The localization and synthesis of some collagen types in developing mouse embryos. Cell 16:953.

Ashhurst DE, Bailey AJ (1980). Locust collagen: morphological and biochemical characterization. Eur J Biochem 103:75.

Bailey AJ, Shellswell GB, Duance VC (1979). Identification and change of collagen types in differentiating myoblasts and developing chick muscle. Nature 278:67.

Bairati A (1972). Collagen: an analysis of phylogenetic aspects. Boll Zool 39:205.

Clément P (1980). Phylogenetic relationships of rotifers, as derived from photoreceptor morphology and other ultrastructural analyses. In Dumont HJ, Green J (eds): "Developments in Hydrobiology 1: Rotatoria," The Hague: DR W Junk BV, p 93.

Cotta-Pereira G, Guerra Rodrigo F, David Ferreira JF (1978). Comparative study between the elastic system fibers in human thin and thick skin. Biol Cell 31:297.

Critchley DR, England MA, Wakely J, Hynes RO (1979). Distribution of fibronectin in the ectoderm of gastrulating chick embryos. Nature 280:498.

Elder HY (1973). Distribution and functions of elastic fibers in the invertebrates. Biol Bull 144:43.

Evans HJ, Sullivan CE, Piez KA (1976). The resolution of Ascaris cuticle collagen into three chain types. Biochem 15:1435.

Franc S (1979). Genèse de la matrice conjonctive de Veretillum cynomorium Pall. (Cnidaires-Anthozoaires). Etude ultrastructurale et autoradiographique. Arch Anat Micr 68:237.

Garrone R (1978). "Phylogenesis of connective tissue. Morphological aspects and biosynthesis of sponge intercellular matrix." Basel: Karger, p 1-250.

Garrone R, Franc JM, Franc S (1979). Les invertebres primitifs (Spongiaires, Cnidaires, Cténaires) ont-ils des membranes basales? Riv Istochim 23: 27.

Garrone R, Lethias C (1980). Caractéristiques membranaires des cellules sphéruleuses (cellules à lectine?) chez l'éponge Chondrosia reniformis Nardo. Biol Cell 38:24a.

Gerisch G (1979). Control circuits in cell aggregation and differentiation of Dictyostelium discoideum. In Ebert JD, Okada TS (eds): "Mechanisms of cell changes", New York: John Wiley and Sons, p 225.

Hay ED (1973). Origin and role of collagen in the embryo. Amer Zool 13:1085.

Hernandez-Nicaise ML, Amsellem J (1980). Ultrastructure of the giant smooth muscle fibre of the Ctenophore Beroe ovata. J Ultrastruct Res (in press).

Hofmann H, Fietzek PP, Kühn K (1980). Comparative analysis of the sequences of the three collagen chains $\alpha_1(I)$, α_2 and $\alpha_1(III)$. Functional and genetic aspects. J Mol Biol 141:293.

Hunt S (1970). "Polysaccharide-protein complexes in invertebrates." London: Acad Press, p 1-321.

Jimenez SA, Bashey RI, Benditt M, Yankowski R (1977). Identification of collagen $\alpha_1(I)$ trimer in embryonic chick tendons and calvaria. Bioc Bioph Res Communic 78:1354.

Kimura S, Matsuura F (1974). The chain composition of several invertebrate collagens. J Biochem 75:1231.

Kimura S, Tanze ML (1977). Nereis cuticle collagen: isolation and characterization of two distinct subunits. Biochem 16:2554.

Labat-Robert J, Pavans de Ceccatty M, Robert L, Auger C, Lethias C, Garrone R (1979). Surface glycoproteins of sponge cells: presence of a fibronectin-like protein on differentiated sponge cell membranes, its role in cell aggregation. In Schauer R (ed): "Glycoconjugates." Stuttgart: Georg Thieme p 431.

Ledger P, Franc S (1978). Calcification of the collagenous axial skeleton of Veretillum cynomorium. Cell Tissue Res 192:249.

Leivo I, Vaheri A, Timpl R, Wartiovaara J (1980). Appearance and distribution of collagens and laminin in the early mouse embryo. Develop Biol 76:100.

Linsenmayer TF, Toole BP, Trelstad RL (1973). Temporal and spatial transitions in collagen types during embryonic chick limb development. Develop Biol 35:232.

Locke M, Huie P (1975). Staining of the elastic fibers in insect connective tissue after tannic acid/glutaraldehyde fixation. Tissue and Cell 7:211.

Low FN (1967). Developing boundary (basement) membranes in the chick embryo. Anat Rec 159:231.

Mathews MB (1975). "Connective tissue. Macromolecular structure and evolution". Berlin: Springer-Verlag, p 1-318.

Mayne R, Vail MS, Miller EJ (1975). Analysis of changes in collagen biosynthesis that occur when chick chondrocytes are grown in 5-bromo-2-deoxyuridine. Proc Nat Acad Sci 72:4511.

Monsigny M, Kieda C, Roche AC (1979). Membrane lectins. Biol Cell 35:289.

Müller W, Zahn R, Kurelec B, Müller I, Uhlenbruck G, Vaith P (1979). Aggregation of sponge cells. A novel mechanism of controlled intercellular adhesion, basing on the interrelation between glycosyltransferases and glycosidases.

J Biol Chem 254:1280.

Norwig A, Nowack, Hieber-Rogall E (1973). Sea anemone collagen: further evidence for the existence of only one α-chain type. J Molec Evol 2:175.

Person P, Philpott DE (1969). The nature and significance of invertebrate cartilages. Biol Rev 44:1.

Pucci-Minafra I, Galante R, Minafra S (1978). Identification of collagen in the Aristotle's lanternae of Paracentrotus lividus. J Submicr Cytol 10:53.

Reddi AH (1976). Collagen and cell differentiation. In Ramachandran G, Reddi AH (eds): "Biochemistry of collagen", New York: Plenum Press, p 449.

Sage EH, Gray WR (1977). Evolution of elastic structure. In Sandberg L, Gray W, Franzblau C (eds): "Elastin and Elastic Tissue", New York: Plenum Press, p 291.

Slavkin H, Greulich R (1975). "Extracellular matrix influences on gene expression". New York: Acad Press, p 1-833.

Vaheri A, Ruoslahti E, Mosher D (1978). Fibroblast surface protein. Ann N Y Acad Sci 312:1.

Van de Vyver G (1979). Cellular mechanisms of recognition among sponges. In Lévi C, Boury-Esnault N (eds): "Sponge Biology", Paris: C.N.R.S., p 195.

Von der Mark H, Von der Mark K (1978). αA(αB)2 collagen: a specific biochemical marker for muscle differentiation. In Robert L (ed): "Biochemistry of normal and pathological connective tissues", Paris: C.N.R.S., p 214.

Von de Mark H, Von der Mark K, Gay S (1976). Study of differential collagen synthesis during development of the chick embryo by immunofluorescence. Develop Biol 48:237.

Von der Mark K, Von der Mark H, Timpl R, Trelstad RL (1977). Immunofluorescent localization of collagen types I, II and III in the embryonic chick eye. Develop Biol 59:75.

Connective Tissue Research:
Chemistry, Biology, and Physiology, Pages 151–162
© **1981 Alan R. Liss, Inc., 150 Fifth Avenue, New York, N.Y. 10011**

INTERACTIONS BETWEEN CONNECTIVE TISSUE COMPONENTS

Vladimír Podrazký

Research Institute of Food Industry,
Prague, Czechoslovakia.

INTRODUCTION

The interactions which occur among the connective tissue
components are an excellent example on the self-assembly of a
system by means of non-covalent binding. The physical characteristics of connective tissue are greatly dependent on the
interrelationships of the high-molecular weight components in
their specific milieu. However, in spite of the system being
of very complex nature and including a number of substances,
the study of the interactions of the connective tissue high-
molecular weight components has, with a few exceptions, not
yet advanced beyond binary systems.

The main attention has been paid to the interaction between the two major connective tissue components, collagen on
side and proteoglycans or their constituents, i.e. glycosaminoglycans and protein core, on the other. More recently,
much interest has focused on studies involving proteoglycan
subunits, link proteins and hyaluronic acid which give rise
to proteoglycan complexes. Comparatively little concern has
been given to the interaction of collagen with structural
glycoproteins although it has been suggested that glycoproteins may have a function in maintaining the structural
stability of collagen fibrils (Jackson and Bentley, 1968) and
in controlling the collagen fibril diameter (Anderson et al.,
1977). On the other hand, the interaction between cell
surface glycoprotein and collagen is now under detailed study
due to its putative importance in the cell-to-cell and cell-
to-matrix attachment.

The other fibrillar protein of connective tissue, elastin, has been studied only negligibly from the point of view of its interactions with other connective tissue high-molecular weight components although it seems that such inter-actions, especially those with glycoproteins, are associated with the early stages of elastogenesis (Robert et al., 1971).

The present contribution deals mainly with the inter-action of proteoglycans or their constituents with collagen in terms of the nature of the interaction, and of the effect of the interaction on the collagen fibrillogenesis. Further, the interaction of proteoglycans with elastin will be briefly mentioned.

NATURE OF THE PROTEOGLYCAN-COLLAGEN INTERACTION

The proteoglycan subunit consists of a protein core with laterally attached glycosaminoglycan chains (Hascall and Riolo, 1972). Much basic information on its reactivity may be gained, consequently, from the study of the properties of the glycosaminoglycan chains alone.

The first observation on the glycosaminoglycan-collagen interaction was that of Meyer et al. (1937a, 1937b) who found that chondroitin sulphate formed insoluble complexes on inter-action with gelatin. The complex formation was thought to be due to the basic amino groups in gelatin and the sulphate and carboxyl groups in chondroitin sulphate. This early sugges-tion has been confirmed since by a number of others using a variety of methods. It is now generally accepted that co-operative electrostatic binding is the main factor, although not necessarily the only one, in the glycosaminoglycan-collagen interaction which appears to be mediated by ester sulphate groups on the glycosaminoglycan molecule and lysyl and arginyl side chains on the collagen molecule (Podrazký et al., 1971). One molecule of glycosaminoglycan bears a great number of sulphate groups which are distributed along the whole polysaccharide chain. On the other hand, the content of lysyl and arginyl residues in collagen is approxi-mately only 8% of the total amino acid residues. Moreover, the polar amino acid residues are accumulated in clusters along the collagen molecule. This is the reason why the number of reactive sites on a collagen molecule is restricted as pointed out by Öbrink and Sundelöf (1973). They found that complexes of collagen and chondroitin sulphate or

dermatan sulphate contained 2, 4 or 5 moles of glycosaminoglycan per one mole of collagen. In a later work (Öbrink et
al., 1975), a minimum of three binding sites for chondroitin-
4-sulphate was found on the collagen molecule with different
affinities to the polysaccharide. While two of them were
able to bind chondroitin-4-sulphate chains of any molecular
weight, the third one had no affinity to low-molecular weight
chains. The presumption that further binding sites on the
collagen molecule may exist for high-molecular weight glycosaminoglycans is supported by the previously mentioned results.
But in spite of the regular distribution of charged groups
in glycosaminoglycans, they, too, seem to bear only a limited
number of binding sites available for collagen. In the excess
of collagen, one molecule of dermatan sulphate is able to
combine with a maximum of five collagen molecules (Öbrink
and Sundelöf, 1973).

It was postulated by Mathews (1970) that the undenatured
state of collagen is required for its interaction with
chondroitin sulphate. In accordance with this, no complex
formation could be detected between proteoglycan and denatured tropocollagen by isoelectrofocusing (Podrazký and
Steven, unpublished results). It may be of interest to note
that this behaviour is in a sharp contrast to the collagen-
fibronectin interaction which is weak with native collagen
but very strong with denatured collagen (Jilek and Hörmann,
1979). There are certain differences between the collagen
types in their binding to glycosaminoglycans or proteoglycans.
While type I collagen has a higher activity than type II
collagen as regards the interaction with proteoglycan subunit
(Lee-Own and Anderson, 1976), there is a preferential binding
of proteoglycans to α_2 chain or β_{12} component of type I
collagen (Lee-Own and Anderson, 1975), which can be explained
either in terms of a more basic nature of the α_2 chain as
compared to the α_1 chain, or by a more favourable spatial
arrangement of the basic amino acid residues in the α_2 chain.

Toole (1976) compared the binding capacity to proteoglycan of collagen types I, II and III and determined the
ratios of proteoglycan to collagen in aggregates formed in
the excess of proteoglycan. He found the molar ratios of
1:16, 1:7 and 1:22 for collagen types I, II and III, respectively.

On the part of glycosaminoglycans, the extent and strength of their binding to collagen is dependent on several factors.

As the binding is mainly due to electrostatic forces, the net charge and charge density play an important role. Different glycosaminoglycans, consequently, have different binding capacities to collagen. As a rule, those glycosaminoglycans that carry a higher negative charge per a disaccharide unit interact more strongly with collagen. Öbrink (1973a) observed no binding of hyaluronic acid or keratan sulphate to collagen which suggests that the presence of only one negative charge per a disaccharide unit is not sufficient to induce binding even if the charge is provided by the sulphate group which is necessary for the interaction (Gelman and Blackwell, 1973). Consequently, a minimum of two charges per a disaccharide unit is an essential prerequisite. However, while the inability of hyaluronic acid and keratan sulphate to combine with collagen was confirmed e.g. by Greenwald et al. (1975), there exist also contradictory results. Gelman and Blackwell (1974) found that at acid pH the extent of interaction with collagen is greater for hyaluronic acid than for chondroitin 4-sulphate. On the other hand, in experiments with model basic homopeptides, poly-L-lysine and poly-L-arginine, the strength of interaction with glycosaminoglycans was lowest for hyaluronic acid (Gelman et al., 1974). The binding of hyaluronic acid to collagen was observed also by Cundall et al. (1979). Other factors apart from electrostatic forces, however, must be taken into account such as molecular entanglement or entropic interaction.

Another important factor on the glycosaminoglycan side appears to be the spatial distribution of the charged groups. Chondroitin 6-sulphate and chondroitin 4-sulphate revealed a marked difference in their effect on the conformation of poly-L-lysine which was at least 80% helical on the interaction with chondroitin 6-sulphate and only 20% helical on that with chondroitin 4-sulphate (Gelman and Blackwell, 1973). The stoichiometry of the interaction, however, was the same for both chondroitin sulphates. The difference in the strength of binding was attributed to the ability of the sulphate group bearing side chain in chondroitin 6-sulphate to be extended away from the main chain. On the other hand, the exposed position of the sulphate group in chondroitin 6-sulphate renders the interaction with polypeptides more susceptible to the effect of ionic strength (Schodt et al., 1976). A similar stoichiometry for chondroitin 4- and 6-sulphates in their binding to collagen was found also by Cundall et al. (1979). Accordingly, it is the strength of binding and the stability of the complexes under various conditions which manifest the effect of the position of the sulphate group.

The importance of the glycosaminoglycan conformation is stressed by the fact that those glycosaminoglycans that contain L-iduronic acid, i.e. dermatan sulphate and heparan sulphate, have a higher affinity towards collagen than those containing D-glucuronic acid only, even in case of identical charge density and similar molecular weights (Obrink, 1973a). It seems that an important factor is the distance between the anionic groups in the disaccharide unit and, consequently, the charge distribution (Gelman and Blackwell, 1974). In chondroitin 4-sulphate the sulphate and carboxyl groups are located close together which is not the case with dermatan sulphate. Thus, the interaction between collagen and glycosaminoglycans seems to be stronger if the acidic groups in the latter are more separated.

The molecular weight of glycosaminoglycans also plays a certain role in the binding capacity (Obrink and Wasteson, 1971). However, even low-molecular weight fragments of the glycosaminoglycan chains are able to bind ionically to tropocollagen molecule (Podrazký et al., 1971).

Similarly to glycosaminoglycans, the reactivity of the proteoglycan subunit can be expected to reside mainly in the sulphate groups of the polysaccharide chains. For steric reasons, however, only those sulphate groups which are located at or near the ends of the individual chains will be available for the electrostatic interaction. The reactivity of the sulphate groups situated inside the molecule is considerably lowered even for low-molecular weight substances, as compared to the reactivity of the sulphate groups of the separate glycosaminoglycan chains (Podrazký et al., 1971). The reactivity of the proteoglycan subunit will be further influenced by the protein moiety. The protein core protruding from the proteoglycan molecule represents a potential site for additional interactions different from those of glycosaminoglycan chains. Schodt and Blackwell (1976), however, claim that the strength of interaction of poly(L-arginine) with proteoglycans is the same as that with the component polysaccharides as judged from the thermal stability of the products. This conclusion, however, need not be valid for the collagen-proteoglycan interaction as shown in other studies referred to in the following.

The binding of proteoglycan to collagen was reported to be stronger than that of glycosaminoglycans (Greenwald et al., 1975; Oegema et al., 1975). The content of chondroitin sulphate chains in the proteoglycan molecule does not exert any marked influence on the strength of interaction which suggests that the protein core is significantly involved in the complex formation and that its binding to collagen is stronger than the binding of chondroitin sulphate chains (Greenwald et al., 1975). The protein core is bound also to collagen fibrils during their formation although it is not bound as strongly as the intact proteoglycan (Oegema et al., 1975). The strength of the binding of the protein core is dependent on ionic strength. Toole (1976) suggested that the primary specific binding site for collagen is located in the protein core and that the reaction results in a spatial ar-rangement which maximizes electrostatic interaction between chondroitin sulphate chains and collagen with the ensuing aggregate formation. The participation of protein core in the proteoglycan-collagen interaction was suggested also by Gelman et al. (1974) on the basis of the interaction of proteoglycan and its fragments with basic homopolypeptides. They observed a conformation-directing effect between protein core and basic polypeptides.

It should be noted in this connection that proteoglycan complex affects fibrillogenesis of collagen approximately in the same way as the proteoglycan subunit (Oegema et al., 1975). This fact raises some doubts about the postulated primary importance of the protein core in the interaction with collagen because the protein core in the proteoglycan complex is engaged in binding to hyaluronic acid and hence it is not available for the binding to collagen.

INFLUENCE OF GLYCOSAMINOGLYCANS AND PROTEOGLYCANS ON COLLAGEN FIBRILLOGENESIS

Although the ability to form fibrils is an inherent property of monomeric collagen (Gross et al., 1955), it was suggested (Gross, 1956) that glycosaminoglycans might affect the organization of collagen fibrils. The influence of glycosaminoglycans and/or proteoglycans on the collagen fibril formation has been confirmed since in a number of studies.

The study of the kinetics of the collagen fibrillation (Gross and Kirk, 1958; Bensusan and Hoyt, 1958; Wood and Keech, 1960) revealed two distinct phases: the lag phase or nucleation phase during which no increase in turbidity of collagen solutions takes place, and the growth phase in which a rapid increase in turbidity occurs. The nucleation phase and the growth phase appear to be connected, respectively, with the linear and lateral growth of collagen aggregates (Silver and Trelstad, 1979). The kinetic parameters show that both these phases can be influenced if glycosaminoglycans or proteoglycans are present. Glycosaminoglycans, however, greatly differ in their effects and may retard or accelerate collagen fibre formation and modify the width of collagen fibrils in the dependence on their structure and molecular size (Wood, 1960; Keech, 1961; Obrink, 1973b). It is difficult to correlate the influence of glycosaminoglycans on collagen fibrillation with the strength of their binding to collagen because other molecular forces may be involved as already mentioned, such as steric exclusion effect with a consequent increase in the activity of collagen as shown by Obrink (1973b) for the collagen-hyaluronic acid system. The thermal stability of collagen fibrils was not found to be altered by the interaction with glycosaminoglycans (Snowden and Swann, 1980).

In terms of the possible implication in fibrillogenesis in vivo glycosaminoglycans, however, are probably of minor importance compared to proteoglycans which are the prevailing form of the occurence of glycosaminoglycans in tissues (Anderson and Sajdera, 1971). The end-to-end elongation of linear aggregates of collagen which occurs in the lag phase can be markedly retarded though not inhibited in the presence of proteoglycans. On the other hand, if proteoglycans are present only in the growth phase, they do not retard the fibril formation but still do bind to collagen and modify the final organization of fibrils (Oegema et al., 1975). Proteoglycans slightly decrease the thermal stability of collagen which may be the result of the interference with the electrostatic interaction between collagen molecules (Snowden and Swann, 1980). The simplest model for the complex formed between proteoglycans and tropocollagen consists of proteoglycan molecules linked by tropocollagen molecules (Öbrink, 1973a). Still, it must be stressed again that the interaction between the two macromolecular species is of complex nature, and that apart from ionic interactions, entropic interactions (Meyer et al., 1971), steric exclusion and molecular entanglement are probably effective.

Possibly the most convincing evidence in favour of the effect of proteoglycans on the organization of collagen fibres was obtained from the studies concerning the composition and characteristics of the individual parts of the eye (Borcherding et al., 1975). The central cornea is marked by a high concentration of proteoglycans containing keratan sulphate as the major glycosaminoglycan component, and at the same time by a remarkable uniformity of fibre diameter and lamellar arrangement. Distally from the central cornea, this uniformity is gradually lost, the diameter of collagen fibres increases while the total concentration of proteoglycans decreases as well as the proportion of keratan sulphate which is partially replaced by chondroitin sulphate and dermatan sulphate. Thus, morphology of various types of connective tissue may be greatly dependent on the relationships which collagen and proteoglycans bear to one another.

PROTEOGLYCAN-ELASTIN INTERACTION

Similarly to collagen, elastin has an inherent capability of forming fibrils in the absence of other high-molecular weight substances. The aggregation of soluble elastin is directed by hydrophobic interactions as can be expected on the basis of the high content of apolar amino acid residues in this protein. Wood (1958) described the formation of insoluble elastin structures from soluble degradation products of mature elastin under conditions which enabled extensive hydrophobic interactions to take place. Cox et al. (1973) observed under suitable conditions fibre formation both from α-elastin, a high-molecular weight degradation product of elastin, and from the native precursor, tropoelastin (Cox et al., 1974), in the absence of any other high-molecular weight connective tissue component.

A very low content of polar amino acids in elastin suggests that the ionic interactions may be of minor importance, if any, in the elastin fibrillogenesis. On the other hand, it is obvious that the precursor molecule once formed enters an environment of pH value below its isoelectric point in which its basic amino acid residues are ionized and capable of electrostatic interactions. An evidence has been presented that as a result of the interaction with proteoglycans α-elastin undergoes conformational changes towards an increased content of α-helix (Podrazký et al., 1975). Further, it was shown that proteoglycans induce elastin fibril formation by ionic interaction from both α-elastin (Podrazký and Adam, 1975) and tropoelastin (Adam and Podrazký, 1976). The scarcity of experimental observations, however, does not allow at present to decide whether or not ionic interactions with proteoglycans play a part in the elastin fibrillogenesis and may thus have any physiological significance.

CONCLUSION

The physical properties of connective tissues are dependent mainly on the two major extracellular high-molecular weight constituents, collagen and proteoglycans. These macromolecular compounds are capable of electrostatic interaction under physiological conditions. If the interaction takes place during collagen fibrillation, it results in a modification of the size and organization of collagen fibrils. Sufficient line of evidence exists for the presumption that the organization of collagen fibres in vivo may be altered in relation to the structure and amounts of the proteoglycans present.

Adam M, Podrazký V (1976). Fibrillation of tropoelastin induced by proteoglycan. Experientia 32:430.

Anderson HC, Sajdera SW (1971). The fine structure of bovine nasal cartilage. Extraction as a technique to study proteoglycans and collagen in cartilage matrix. J Cell Biol 49:650.

Anderson JC, Labedz RI, Kewley MA (1977). The effect of bovine tendon glycoprotein on the formation of fibrils from collagen solutions. Biochem J 167:345.

Bensusan HB, Hoyt BL (1958). The effect of various parameters on the rate of formation of fibers from collagen solutions. J Am Chem Soc 80:719.

Borcherding MS, Blacik LJ, Sittig RA, Bizzell JW, Breen M, Weinstein HG (1975). Proteoglycans and collagen fibre organization in human corneoscleral tissue. Exp Eye Res 21:59.

Cox BA, Starcher BC, Urry DW (1973). Coacervation of α-elastin results in fiber formation. Biochim Biophys Acta 317:209.

Cox BA, Starcher BC, Urry DW (1974). Coacervation of tropo-elastin results in fiber formation. J Biol Chem 249:997.

Cundall RB, Lawton JB, Murray D, Phillips GO (1979). Poly-electrolyte complexes. 2. Interaction between collagen and polyanions. Int J Biolog Macromolecules 1:215.

Gelman RA, Blackwell J (1973). Mucopolysaccharide-poly-peptide interactions: effect of the position of the sulfate group. Biochim Biophys Acta 297:452.

Gelman RA, Blackwell J (1974). Collagen-mucopolysaccharide interactions at acid pH. Biochim Biophys Acta 342:254.

Gelman RA, Blackwell J, Mathews MB (1974). Interaction of an intact proteoglycan and its fragments with basic homo-polypeptides in dilute aqueous solutions. Biochem J 141: 445.

Greenwald RA, Schwartz CE, Cantor JO (1975). Interaction of cartilage proteoglycans with collagen-substituted agarose gels. Biochem J 145:601.

Gross J (1956). Behavior of collagen units as a model in morphogenesis. J Biophys Biochem Cytol, Suppl 2:261.

Gross J, Highberger JH, Schmitt FO (1955). Extraction of collagen from connective tissue by neutral salt solutions. Proc Natl Acad Sci USA 41:1.

Gross J, Kirk D (1958). The heat precipitation of collagen from neutral salt solutions: Some rate-regulating factors. J Biol Chem 233:355.

Hascall VC, Riolo RL (1972). Characteristics of the protein-keratan sulfate core and of keratan sulfate prepared from bovine nasal cartilage proteoglycan. J Biol Chem 247:4529.

Jackson DS, Bentley HP (1968). Collagen-glycosaminoglycan interactions. In Gould BS (ed): "Treatise on Collagen", Vol 2, London: Academic Press, p 189.

Jilek F, Hörmann H (1979). Fibronectin (cold-insoluble globulin). VI. Influence of heparin and hyaluronic acid on the binding of native collagen. Hoppe Seyler's Z Physiol Chem 360:597.

Keech MK (1961). The formation of fibrils from collagen solutions. IV. Effect of mucopolysaccharides and nucleic acids. An electron microscope study. J Biophys Biochem Cytol 9:193.

Lee-Own V, Anderson JC (1975). The isolation of collagen-associated proteoglycan from bovine nasal cartilage and its preferential interaction with α_2-chains of type I collagen. Biochem J 149:57.

Lee-Own V, Anderson JC (1976). Interaction between proteoglycan subunit and type II collagen from bovine nasal cartilage, and the preferential binding of proteoglycan subunit
to type I collagen. Biochem J 153:259.

Mathews MB (1970). The interactions of proteoglycans and
collagen-model systems. In Balazs EA (ed): "Chemistry
and Biology of the Intercellular Matrix", London and New
York: Academic Press, p 1155.

Meyer FA, Comper WD, Preston BN (1971). Model connective
tissue systems. A physical study of gelatin gels containing
proteoglycans. Biopolymers 10:1351.

Meyer K, Palmer JW, Smyth EM (1937a). On glycoproteins. V.
Protein complexes of chondroitin sulfuric acid. J Biol
Chem 119:501.

Meyer K, Smyth EM (1937b). On glycoproteins. VI. The preparation of chondroitin sulfuric acid. J Biol Chem 119:507.

Obrink B (1973a). A study of the interactions between monomeric tropocollagen and glycosaminoglycans. Eur J Biochem
33:387.

Obrink B (1973b). The influence of glycosaminoglycans on
the formation of fibres from monomeric tropocollagen in
vitro. Eur J Biochem 34:129.

Obrink B, Sundelöf L-O (1973). Light scattering in the study
of associating macromolecules. The binding of glycosaminoglycans to collagen. Eur J Biochem 37:226.

Obrink B, Wasteson Å (1971). Nature of the interaction of
Chondroitin 4-sulphate and chondroitin sulphate proteoglycan with collagen. Biochem J 121:227.

Oegema TR, Laidlaw J, Hascall VC, Dziewiatkowski DD (1975).
The effect of proteoglycans on the formation of fibrils
from collagen solutions. Arch Biochem Biophys 170:698.

Podrazký V, Adam M (1975). Fibrillation of α-elastin induced
by proteoglycan. Experientia 31:523.

Podrazký V, Steven FS, Jackson DS, Weiss JB, Leibovich SJ
(1971). Interaction of tropocollagen with protein-poly-
saccharide complexes. An analysis of the ionic groups
responsible for interaction. Biochim Biophys Acta 229:690.

Podrazký V, Stokrová S, Frič I (1975). Elastin-proteoglycan
interaction. Conformational changes of α-elastin induced
by the interaction. Connective Tissue Res 4:51.

Robert B, Szigeti M, Derouette J-C, Robert L (1971). Studies
on the nature of the "microfibrillar" component of elastic
fibers. Eur J Biochem 21:507.

Schodt KP, Blackwell J (1976). Comparison of four proteoglycans in terms of their interactions with poly(L-arginine).
Biopolymers 15:469.

Schodt KP, Gelman RA, Blackwell J (1976). The effect of changes in salt concentration and pH on the interaction between glycosaminoglycans and cationic polypeptides. Biopolymers 15:1965.

Silver FH, Trelstad RL (1979). Linear aggregation and the turbidimetric lag phase: type I collagen fibrillogenesis in vitro. J Theor Biol 81:515.

Snowden JMK, Swann DA (1980). Effect of glycosaminoglycans and proteoglycan on the in vitro assembly and thermal stability of collagen fibrils. Biopolymers 19:767.

Toole BP (1976). Binding and precipitation of soluble collagen by chick embryo cartilage proteoglycan. J biol Chem 251:895.

Wood GC (1958). The reconstitution of elastin from a soluble protein derived from ligamentum nuchae. Biochem J 69:539.

Wood GC (1960). The formation of fibrils from collagen solutions. 3. Effect of chondroitin sulphate and some other naturally occuring polyanions on the rate of formation. Biochem J 75:605.

Wood GC, Keech MK (1960). The formation of fibrils from collagen solutions. 1. The effect of experimantal conditions: Kinetic and electron-microscope studies. Biochem J 75:588.

Connective Tissue Research:
Chemistry, Biology, and Physiology, Pages 163-182
© 1981 Alan R. Liss, Inc., 150 Fifth Avenue, New York, N.Y. 10011

COLLAGEN POLYMORPHISM IN RELATION TO THE ROLE OF COLLAGEN-
INDUCED PLATELET AGGREGATION IN HAEMOSTASIS AND THROMBOSIS

*M.J. Barnes

Strangeways Research Laboratory,
Worts Causeway, Cambridge, U.K.

INTRODUCTION.

It has long been appreciated that extracellular collagen fibres play a vital role in haemostasis by causing the
aggregation of blood platelets following the exposure of the
latter to tissue collagen as a consequence of injury to the
blood vessel wall. Wharton-Jones for example over a century
ago (1851), whilst studying the circulation in the web of a
frog's foot, observed upon inflicting injury by 'pressing
the web over an artery or vein - a large vein especially -
pretty firmly with a blunt point' what he described as 'a
conglomeration of colourless corpuscles... held together,
apparently, by coagulated fibrin' which formed on the wall
of the vessel and 'more or less completely obstructed it
(the vessel)' at the site of injury. This must represent
one of the earliest observations of platelets aggregating in
response to damage to the vessel wall. Collagen was subsequently identified as the active constituent in the extracellular matrix responsible for the aggregation of platelets
and its activity towards platelets was successfully demonstrated in vitro using suspensions of isolated fibres (Bounameaux, 1959; Hugues, 1960; Kjaerheim and Hovig, 1962;
Zucker and Borelli, 1962; Hovig, 1963).

The clumping together of platelets caused by collagen
serves to form the initial haemostatic plug. Concomitantly
with platelet aggregation coagulation occurs most likely as
a consequence of the activity of 'tissue factor' (thrombo-
plastin) which is released from injured tissues and is able
to initiate the extrinsic pathway of coagulation.
*External Staff Member of the Medical Research Council.

Coagulation itself of course contributes directly to the arrest of bleeding and at the same time fibrin produced as the end-product of the coagulation sequence of reactions serves to reinforce the platelet plug. The subject of haemostasis has been reviewed by Thomas (1977) and Zucker (1980).

In addition to its role in haemostasis through the induction of platelet aggregation, collagen may also be involved in promoting the coagulation process, either directly by induction of the intrinsic pathway of coagulation through activation of factor XII (Niewiarowski et al., 1966; Wilner et al., 1968) but more likely perhaps, since the former reaction is disputed (Zacharski & Rosenstein, 1977), indirectly through its action on platelets, causing the release or exposure of platelet-bound coagulation factors which may subsequently be relocated on the surface of the platelet and which are able to contribute to the coagulation process. Thus stimulation of platelets by collagen has been reported to yield activated factor XI associated with the platelets (Walsh, 1972). This particular response to collagen stimulation has however been questioned (Osterud, 1979). Collagen has been shown more certainly to cause an increase in platelet factor V activity. Osterud and co-workers in their studies (Osterud et al., 1977) have concluded that collagen induces conformational changes on the surface of the platelet that results in the binding to the surface of plasma factor V. In addition it is thought, collagen causes the 'exposure' of activated factor V already contained within the platelet.

As must then be apparent in some degree from the foregoing there exists an intimate relationship between the two processes of platelet aggregation and coagulation serving ultimately to effect haemostasis; the one process can assist or augment the other and collagen may play a key role in both. Thus collagen not only stimulates platelets to aggregate but also in so doing facilitates the onset of coagulation at the site of bleeding by rendering platelet-bound coagulation factors, such as factor V already mentioned, factor VIII and fibrinogen available to the coagulation cascade of reactions. Factor VIII not only participates in coagulation but also appears to facilitate platelet binding to collagen (Baumgartner et al., 1980). Fibrinogen, converted to fibrin in coagulation, is also essential for the actual platelet aggregatory mechanism. The process of

coagulation yields thrombin which not only converts fibrinogen to fibrin but can also stimulate platelets thereby causing further platelet aggregation at the point of injury.
Fibrin as already stipulated, besides its role in coagulation can also act to stabilize the platelet clump. These
various interactions all serve to promote aggregation and
coagulation most effectively at the site of injury and to
prevent their occurrence elsewhere.

During the stimulation of platelets by collagen culmin-
ating in platelet aggregation a complex sequence of events
is initiated within the platelet the precise relationship
between which has still to be fully elucidated (Gordon,
1976). Following their exposure to collagen fibres, platelets first attach to the collagen surface, the process known
as platelet adhesion. During this attachment, platelets
undergo a change in shape, spreading flat upon the fibre
surface. Platelets then undergo the process of degranulation
(the 'release reaction') during which they secrete specific
granule products such as the coagulation proteins already
alluded to and the substance adenosine diphosphate (ADP)
which is a highly potent platelet stimulatory agent (Zucker,
1980). At the same time, arachidonate is liberated from
membrane-bound phospholipids and is converted by the aspirin-
sensitive enzyme cyclo-oxygenase to endoperoxides which are
then converted to specific prostaglandins, and most impor-
tantly the compound thromboxane A_2 (TXA_2). The latter is a
very active vasoconstrictor (a property that further aids
the haemostatic process) and a very powerful stimulator of
platelet secretion and aggregation (Moncada and Vane, 1978;
Moncada and Amezcua, 1979; Mustard et al., 1980). As a
consequence of this series of reactions neighnouring platelets become stimulated and attach to those already adherent
to the collagen surface, and then to each other, the process
known as platelet aggregation. The relative contribution of
ADP and TXA_2 to the overall aggregation process is still
uncertain (Lages and Weiss, 1980). It has been considered
that TXA_2 acts to cause the release of ADP which can be
regarded as the actual aggregatory agent (See Claesson and
Malmsten, 1977). ADP (plus fibrinogen as co-factor), unlike
collagen, is known to be able to cause aggregation directly -
primary aggregation - independently of platelet secretion and
prostaglandin synthesis. However it has also been maintained
that the release of ADP is not sufficient to account entirely
for all the aggregation (Nunn, 1979). Furthermore there
is evidence that TXA_2 can induce aggregation in the absence

of secretion and therefore independently of ADP (Charo et al., 1977).

Arising from its involvement in haemostasis, collagen may also play an important part in thrombosis which can be regarded as the pathological expression of haemostasis and the occurrence of which may result in death through heart failure, a stroke or some other cause. Platelet aggregation induced by collagen in the vessel wall is thought, as in haemostasis, to play a central role, at least in some forms of the disease. For a consideration of various aspects of thrombosis, the reader is referred to the recent publications by Thomas (1978), Nordoy (1979) and Wall and Harker (1980).

The activation of platelets by collagen may also be an important early event in atherosclerosis. In this disease, it is postulated (Ross and Glomset, 1976) that damage to or loss of vascular endothelium results in the exposure of subendothelial constituents to circulating platelets which are stimulated to release a peptide, platelet-derived growth factor, which causes the proliferation of smooth muscle cells migrating into the intimal region at the site where endothelial damage or loss has occurred. As a result the atherosclerotic plaque is formed. The proliferating smooth muscle cells produce new extracellular matrix which contributes to the occlusion of the vessel lumen by the plaque. Plasma lipoproteins (particularly LDL) become deposited within the fibrous lesion which eventually proceeds to the so-called complicated form displaying calcification, ulceration and thrombus formation.

In the vessel wall, endoperoxides arising from arachidonate are converted not into TXA_2 but the prostaglandin, PGI_2 (prostacyclin). This compound is a potent inhibitor of platelet secretion and aggregation and can induce the disaggregation of pre-existing aggregates (Moncada and Vane, 1978; Moncada and Amezcua, 1979). It is considered a balance exists between the production of PGI_2 by the vessel wall on the one hand and TXA_2 by platelets on the other, the disturbance of which may be of critical importance in the pathogenesis of thrombosis and arterial disease.

So far in this article collagen has been referred to in the sense of occurring as a single protein. However, with the advent of collagen polymorphism and the recognition

of the existence of a family of genetically-distinct collagen subtypes, such a view is no longer tenable and it is
necessary to reconsider the involvement of collagen in haemostasis and the pathological processes of thrombosis and
atherosclerosis in the light of its known polymorphism.
Several studies have now been directed at the question of
the comparative platelet reactivity of the different collagen subtypes and this subject will be considered below.
For a more general consideration of the collagen-platelet
interaction, the reader is referred to the recent reviews
by Jaffe (1976), Gastpar et al., (1978), Beachey et al.,
(1979) and Barnes (1980).

COLLAGEN POLYMORPHISM IN THE BLOOD VESSEL WALL.

     Following the initial observations of Chung and
Miller (1974) and Trelstad (1974) it is now well established
that the large vessel wall contains two different interstitial collagens referred to as collagen types I and III. In
comparison to most other tissues, type III collagen occurs
in the vessel wall in relatively large amounts. Immunofluorescent studies have shown the occurrence of this collagen in the media in close association with the elastic
laminae, type I being located more in the spaces between the
laminae (Gay et al., 1975; McCullagh et al., 1980). At
least in the young vessel wall where there is little if any
intimal thickening and the intima consists essentially of
endothelium with its underlying basement membrane, type III
collagen has been detected in the total absence of type I
in the space between the basement membrane and the internal
elastic lamina. Because of this, this particular collagen
has been considered to be of especial importance in thrombosis (Gay et al., 1975). However, the intima exhibits a
widespread thickening with increasing age and the author
and his colleagues (M.J. Barnes and L.F. Morton, unpublished
data) have detected, by biochemical analysis, type I collagen in the diffusely thickened intima in appreciable greater
quantity than type III. Similarly type I collagen has been
reported to be in excess relative to type III in the atherosclerotic intimal plaque (McCullagh and Balian, 1975).
The possible involvement of type I collagen in thrombus
formation cannot therefore be disregarded.

     The two basement membrane-associated collagens, types
IV and V, have also been detected in the vessel wall. It is

likely that each of these collagens is located in both the
intimal subendothelial basement membrane as well as that
associated with the medial smooth-muscle cell. Their
occurrence in the subendothelial basement membrane could be
regarded as of particular significance in relation to
thrombosis. Trelstad (1974) has detected type IV collagen
in human aorta by biochemical analysis. Chung et al.,
(1976) have reported the presence of collagen type V in the
media of the vessel wall but in a form comprised of B-chains
only. Neither A nor B chains related to type V collagen
could be detected in the intima. These observations seem to
support the contention that so-called Type V is really two
collagens of chain composition A_2 and B_2 respectively.
However, the author and his colleagues (M.J. Barnes and
L.F. Morton, unpublished data) have detected chains of both
A and B type in the media and in the thickened intima.
There appeared to be a substantial amount of type V (relative to the interstitial collagens) in the latter in comparison to the media. The ratio of B:A was found to be
close to 2:1 in both intima and media preparations which
may support the view more that type V is a single collagen
of chain composition B_2A. Type V collagen has been detected
in intima and media by immunofluorescent techniques using
antibodies directed against a type V preparation of composition B_2A. The distribution observed supported the notion
of this collagen as a basement membrane-type but there was
also evidence for its location in some degree outside basement membrane structures (McCullagh et al., 1980).

A further collagenous species has been identified in
the wall of human aorta. This was initially described by
Chung et al., (1976) who reported the isolation of this new
species as a peptide of 55,000 daltons (following reduction).
The existence of this collagen was confirmed by Furoto and
Miller (1980) who have detected its presence in human placenta. Balleisen and Rauterberg (1980) have isolated a
similar entity from bovine placenta and refer to it as
short-chain (SC) collagen.

There is then a variety of different collagens in the
vessel wall each with a distinct distribution. The interaction of platelets with the vessel wall following injury
will depend therefore on the one hand upon the type(s) of
collagen exposed (which may vary according to the exact
nature of the injury incurred) and on the other upon the
particular platelet reactivity of each individual collagen

within the vessel wall. The platelet reactivity first of
the interstitial collagens and then of the basement membrane-associated collagens will be considered below.

PLATELET REACTIVITY OF THE INTERSTITIAL COLLAGENS.

In the past five years or so, a number of different
groups have made a comparison of the platelet reactivity of
the two interstitial collagens types I and III (Balleisen
et al., 1975; Barnes et al., 1976; Hugues et al., 1976;
Santcro and Cunningham, 1977). In all instances it has been
found that when these two collagens are presented in solution to a suspension of platelets, type III collagen is very
much more active at inducing platelet aggregation than type
I. However, if, prior to the addition to platelets the
solutions are first preincubated at $37^{o}C$ either in platelet-
poor-plasma or a suitable buffer, conditions known to promote collagen fibrillogenesis, then it is observed that the
lag period preceding platelet aggregation is reduced and the
aggregatory activity of each collagen is greatly enhanced.
Both collagens now exhibit a similar order of aggregatory
activity. These general observations are exemplified by the
data of the author and his colleagues (Barnes et al., 1976)
presented in Figures 1 and 2. We found for example, that a
solution of collagen type I (from human aorta) failed to
cause platelet aggregation at a concentration of 60 µg/ml in
contrast to the activity of a solution of type III collagen
(from the same source) measurable at a concentration of
around 5 µg/ml. However after preincubation, both collagens
readily induced platelet aggregation, type III at around
0.5-1.5 µg/ml and type I at around 2-3 µg/ml. Similar observations were made with collagens types I and III from chick
skin. After preincubation type I collagen was at least as
active as Type III. These findings are entirely consistent
with the concept advanced on the basis of earlier studies
with type I collagen that the quaternary structure is of
paramount importance in determining the ability of collagen
to induce platelet aggregation and that collagen can only
exhibit aggregatory activity when in fibrillar form (Muggli
and Baumgartner, 1973; Brass and Bensusan, 1974; Jaffe and
Deykin 1974). The increased activity following preincubation
can be attributed to the formation of fibrils. The reason
for the markedly greater activity of type III collagen (relative to that of type I) when presented to platelets in solution form is unclear but presumably reflects a greater

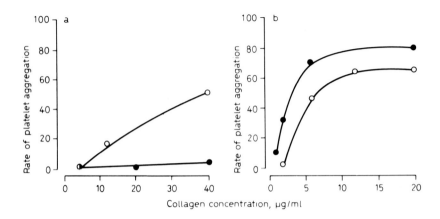

Figure 1.

Platelet aggregation by collagens types I and III from chick skin. Platelet aggregation was measured in 0.1 ml samples of human citrated platelet-rich plasma by observing changes in optical density following the addition of known amounts of collagen. The rate of aggregation was obtained from the maximum rate of change in light transmission. (a) Platelet responses following addition of collagen in solution (10 μl or less) in 0.1 M acetic acid. Open circles = type III; closed circles, type I. (b) Responses following addition of collagens in fibrillar suspension: collagen solutions were preincubated with an equal volume of cell-free plasma. From Barnes et al., (1976) by permission of the Biochemical Journal.

facility on the part of the pepsin-solubilized type III, in comparison to pepsin-treated type I, to form fibrils in platelet-rich plasma at 37°C.

The greater activity of type III collagen solutions in comparison to those of type I led to the proposition (Hugues et al., 1976) that the activity detectable in type I solutions (of sufficiently high concentration) was really attributable to the presence of type III collagen as a contaminant and that type I collagen lacked genuine platelet aggregatory activity. However this notion seems untenable in view of the

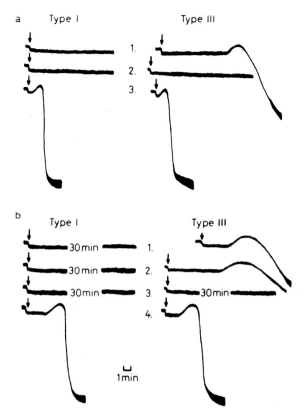

Figure 2.

Platelet aggregation by collagens types I and III from human aorta and chick skin. Platelet aggregation was measured as described in Figure 1. The traces shown represent actual changes in optical transmission following addition of collagen (at the arrow) to a final concentration of 20 μg/ml. (a) Chick collagen: (1) Addition of collagen in solutions in 0.1 M acetic acid, (2) Addition after preincubation in an equal volume of 0.9% sodium chloride; treatment under these conditions yields inactive precipitates. (3) After preincubation in 0.38 M disodium hydrogen phosphate or cell-free plasma; preincubation under these conditions yields highly potent native-type fibrils. (b) Human collagens: (1) As (a) 1. (2) Addition of collagen after preincubation in an equal volume of cell-free plasma; the results suggest an inhibitor of human collagen fibrillogenesis in human plasma. (3) After preincubation in an equal volume of 0.9% sodium chloride. (4) After preincubation in an equal volume of 0.38 M disodium hydrogen phosphate. From Barnes et al. (1976) by permission of the Biochemical Journal.

comparable activity exhibited by each collagen when presented to platelets in fibrillar form. Furthermore, the intrinsic activity of type I collagen has been verified by the demonstration of the platelet reactivity of the collagen, α1(I) trimer (Balleisen et al., 1976; Fauvel et al., 1978). The latter, of chain composition $[α1(I)]_3$, was prepared by isolating α1(I) chains chromatographically (thereby ensuring removal of any contaminating type III chains) and then subjecting the purified chains to conditions which permitted their renaturation to yield type I trimer. The use of monospecific antibodies to inhibit the collagen-platelet interaction has also pointed to the genuine platelet aggregatory activity of type I collagen (Balleisen et al., 1979).

In any event type II cartilage collagen (Balleisen et al., 1975) as well as the basement membrane collagens, types IV and V (see below),have all been shown to be able to induce platelet aggregation. It is clear therefore that this activity is not one attributable to a single specific collagen type. In the author's view fibrils of collagens types I and III occurring in the vessel wall will both possess a highly potent platelet aggregatory activity.

PLATELET REACTIVITY OF BASEMENT MEMBRANE-ASSOCIATED COLLAGENS

In initial studies conducted by the author and his colleagues (Barnes and MacIntyre, 1979a,b) neither type IV collagen (from bovine anterior lens capsule) nor type V (from human placenta or bovine lung) were found to exhibit platelet aggregatory activity even when tested at very high concentration (type IV up to 1000 μg/ml; type V from placenta, up to 750 μg/ml, from bovine lung, up to 200 μg/ml) or after preincubation of solutions at $37^\circ C$, or their dialysis at $4^\circ C$ against 0.02M Na_2HPO_4, treatments both known in the case of the interstitial collagens to yield highly potent fibrils of characteristic 67nm periodicity (as observed by electron microscopy). Trelstad and Carvalho (1979) reported similar observations.

This inactivity of collagens types IV and V could have reflected a basic inability of the basement membrane type of collagen to react with platelets. However, particularly in view of the known importance of the quaternary structure in defining the ability of the interstitial collagens to stimulate platelets, we felt it could also reflect the absence in the type IV and V collagen samples of a suitable fibrillar structure to permit platelet aggregation. The studies of Trelstad and Lawley (1977), for example, suggested that basement membrane-associated collagens failed to yield fibrils of 67nm periodicity when solutions were treated under conditions known to be effective in this respect for the interstitial collagens. In order therefore to be able to test the platelet aggregatory activity of the basement membrane-associated collagens when possessing a defined polymeric structure, we attempted to obtain from solutions of collagens types IV and V,segment-long-spacing (SLS) polymers in which the molecules are assembled laterally in a 'head-to-head' and 'tail-to-tail' alignment. The latter are readily produced from solutions of the interstitial collagens by dialysis against an acidic solution of ATP. We found that collagens IV and V also yield SLS structures under these circumstances (Figure 3). These proved like those of the interstitial collagens to be able to induce platelet aggregation (Barnes et al., 1980). Type IV SLS polymers exhibited an order of activity similar to that of type I SLS aggregates but those of type V exhibited a somewhat lower activity (Figure 4). Prior to testing for platelet aggregatory activity it was necessary to remove ATP. SLS polymers were therefore first stabilized by treatment with formaldehyde prior to the removal of ATP by dialysis. This treatment caused end-to-end assembly of SLS polymers to yield F-SLS (Figure 3) and we consider it may be the latter polymeric species that is actually responsible for the aggregation of platelets. This would be in accord with the conclusion of Wang et al. (1978) that 'single' SLS forms are not able to induce aggregation and that a molecular assembly with a minimal length equivalent to three collagen molecules is required. Some variation in activity we observed from one SLS preparation to another for each type of collagen may be attributable to variation in the degree of end-to-end polymerisation of SLS bundles.

We were subsequently able to produce from a solution of
type V collagen (from human placenta) fibrils of 67nm
periodicity by prolonged dialysis against physiological saline at 25°C (Figure 5). These also proved to be able to
induce platelet aggregation with an order of activity comparable to that of type I fibrils produced in similar manner
(Figure 6). Furthermore we later found that dialysis of a

(a)   **(b)**   **(c)**

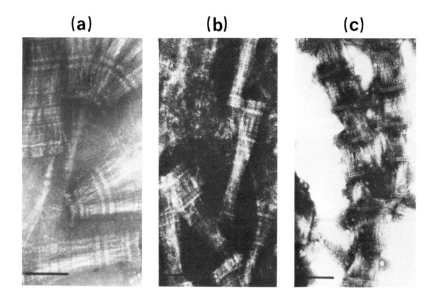

Figure 3.

     Electron micrographs of SLS aggregates of (a) type V
(b) type IV and (c) type I collagen from human placenta.
The type I preparation was examined after treatment with the
cross-linking agent formaldehyde and shows the end-to-end
polymerisation of SLS aggregates into F-SLS form resulting
from this treatment. SLS aggregates of types IV and V
collagens showed similar end-to-end polymerisation when
treated with formaldehyde. The bar represents 0.1 μm in
(a) and (b) and 0.25 μm in (c). From Barnes et al. (1980)
by permission of Thrombosis Research.

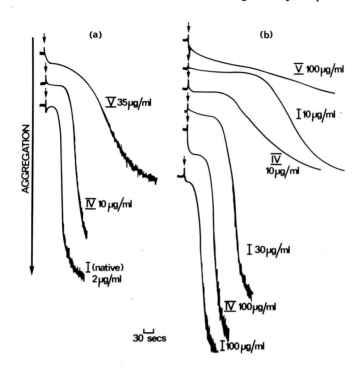

Figure 4.

    Platelet aggregation by SLS polymers of collagens type
I, IV and V. The results of two separate experiments are
shown. Activity was measured at the concentrations specified (a) Aggregation by SLS forms of types IV and V collagens
(from human placenta) and by native-type fibrils of type I
(from bovine tendon) (b) Aggregation by SLS forms of type IV
and V collagens from human placenta and type I from rat tail
tendon (SLS aggregate of type I collagen from human placenta
behaved similarly to those of type I from rat tendon).
From Barnes et al. (1980) by permission of Thrombosis
Research.

solution of type IV collagen (from human placenta but not
other sources apparently) against 0.02M Na$_2$HPO$_4$ at 4°C
yielded non-striated fibrils that exhibited appreciable
platelet aggregatory activity (Figures 5 and 6). Chiang

et al. (1980) have also found that fibrils of 67nm periodicity of type V collagen can induce platelet aggregation and Balleisen and Rauterberg (1980) have reported, in contrast to our findings, that type V collagen solutions can induce platelet aggregation when preincubated in platelet-poor-plasma.

Our results have clearly demonstrated that the basement membrane-associated collagens can induce platelet aggregation if presented to platelets in fibrillar form and that, as stressed already, quaternary structure rather than type per se

(a)   **(b)**   **(c)**

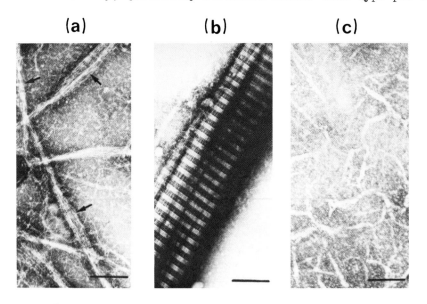

Figure 5.

(a) and (b) Electron micrograph of fibrils of type V collagen (from human placenta) obtained by dialysis of a solution against physiological saline at 25°C. Some fibrils appeared 'loosely-formed' with striations first becoming visable (as in (a) where examples are arrowed) whilst others appeared (as in (b)) with well-defined striations comparable to the native-type fibril of the interstitial collagens, with a 67nm periodicity. (c) Non-striated fibrils of type IV collagen (from human placenta) formed by dialysis of a solution against 0.02M Na_2HPO_4. The bar represents 0.25µm. From Barnes et al. (1980) by permission of Thrombosis Research.

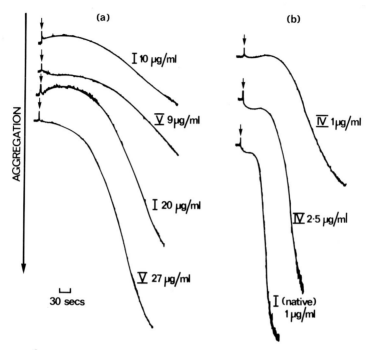

Figure 6.

Platelet aggregation by: (a) type I and type V collagen fibrils of 67nm periodicity formed by dialysis of solutions of these collagens from human placenta against physiological saline at 25°C; (b) non-striated fibrils of type IV collagen (from human placenta) formed by dialysis of a solution against 0.02M Na$_2$HPO$_4$ compared to native-type fibrils of type I (from bovine tendon). Activity was measured at the concentrations specified. From Barnes et al. (1980) by permission of Thrombosis Research.

determines the ability of any particular collagen to induce aggregation. Furthermore our results indicate that the native-type fibril of 67nm periodicity characteristic of the interstitial collagens is not an obligatory structural requirement for aggregation. The activity we observed with non-striated fibrils of type IV collagen implies further that a high degree of order in assembly is not in itself essential.

Nevertheless the native-type fibril of 67nm periodicity
appears to be the most potent polymeric species. The most
active preparation the author and his colleagues (Barnes et
al., 1980) have tested is a highly-polymerised but highly-
dispersed preparation of native-type fibres obtained directly
from bovine flexor tendon (kindly donated by Ethicon Inc,
Somerville, New Jersey, USA), active at around 0.2 µg/ml.

Albeit then the basement membrane-associated collagens
are able under suitable conditions in vitro to adopt a
fibrillar structure that can induce platelet aggregation,
it is uncertain how far these collagens exist in vivo in a
polymeric form possessing such activity. Basement membranes
are generally regarded as amorphous structures and certainly
do not appear to contain fibrils of 67nm periodicity. The
platelet reactivity of basement membranes is a question of
some uncertainty. The electron microscopic studies of
Baumgartner and his colleagues (Baumgartner and Muggli, 1976)
have demonstrated the attachment of platelets to the sub-
endothelium when the endothelium is removed experimentally.
Small aggregates are initially formed but these rapidly
disperse leaving essentially a monolayer of adherent platelets. Attachment is thought to occur to the subendothelial
basement membrane and this phenomenon, it is considered,
may be of importance physiologically in assisting the main-
tenance of vascular integrity in the event of detachment of
the endothelium (perhaps during the course of its normal
turnover). Benditt and colleagues (Huang et al., 1974;
Huang and Benditt, 1978) have reported that human glomerular
basement membrane permits platelet adhesion but does not
induce aggregation. The adhesive property is attributed to
a glycoprotein element in the membrane and not to collagen.
Freytag et al. (1978) however have found that bovine glomerular basement membrane induces aggregation and that the
platelet reactivity is attributable to both collagen and
non-collagenous moieties. Balleisen and Rauterberg (1980)
have presented evidence that both type IV collagen and the
recently-described 'short-chain' collagen could be involved
in the adhesion of platelets to basement membrane.

The question of the platelet reactivity of subendothelial basement membrane is of especial significance in relation to thrombosis. How far thrombus formation reflects an
alteration in basement membrane platelet reactivity from
one that normally allows adhesion only or alternatively the
aggregation of platelets by the subendothelial interstitial

collagens rather than collagens of the basement membrane
remains an important issue.

REFERENCES

Balleisen L, Gay S, Marx R, Kühn K (1975). Comparative investigations of the influence of human and bovine collagen
types I, II and III on the aggregation of human platelets.
Klin Wochen 53: 903.

Balleisen L, Marx R, Kühn K (1976). Platelet: collagen interaction: The influence of native and modified collagen
(type I) on the aggregation of human platelets.
Haemostasis 5: 155.

Balleisen L, Nowack H, Gay S, Timpl R (1979). Inhibition of
collagen-induced platelet aggregation by antibodies to
distinct types of collagen. Biochem J 180: 683.

Balleisen L, Rauterberg J (1980). Platelet activation by
basement membrane collagens. Thromb Res 18: 725.

Barnes M J (1980). The collagen-platelet interaction. In
Jayson M I V, Weiss J B (eds): "Collagen in Health and
Disease". London: Churchill Livingstone (in press).

Barnes M J, Bailey A J, Gordon J L, MacIntyre D E (1980).
Platelet aggregation by basement membrane-associated collagens. Thromb Res 18: 375.

Barnes M J, Gordon J L, MacIntyre D E (1976). Platelet-aggre-
gating activity of type I and type III collagens from
human aorta and chicken skin. Biochem J 160: 647.

Barnes M J, MacIntyre D E (1979a). Collagen-induced platelet
aggregation: The activity of basement membrane collagens
relative to other collagen types. Front Matrix Biol 7: 246.

Barnes M J, MacIntyre D E (1979b). Platelet reactivity of
isolated constituents of the blood vessel wall. Haemostasis 8: 158.

Baumgartner H R, Muggli R (1976). Adhesion and aggregation:
morphological demonstration and quantitation in vivo and
in vitro. In Gordon J L (ed): "Platelets in Biology and
Pathology". Amsterdam: Elsevier/North Holland Biomedical
Press, p23.

Baumgartner H R, Tschopp T B, Weiss H J (1980). Shear rate
dependent inhibition of platelet adhesion and aggregation
on collagenous surfaces by antibodies to human factor
VIII/von Willebrand factor. Brit J Haematol 44: 127.

Beachey E H, Chiang T M, Kang A H (1979). Collagen: platelet
interaction. Intern Rev Connect Tiss Res 8: 1.

Bounameaux V (1959). L'accolement des plaquettes fibres sous-
endotheliales. Comp Rend Seances Societe Biol, Paris 153:658.

Brass L F, Bensusan H B (1974). The role of collagen quaternary structure in the platelet: collagen interaction. J Clin Invest 54: 1480.

Charo I F, Feinman R D, Detwiler T C, Smith J B, Ingerman C M, Silver M J (1977). Prostaglandin endoperoxides and thromboxane A_2 can induce platelet aggregation in the absence of secretion. Nature, Lond 269: 66.

Chiang T M, Mainardi C L, Seyer J M, Kang A H (1980). Collagen: Platelet interaction. Type V (A-B) collagen induces platelet aggregation. J Lab Clin Med 95: 99.

Chung E, Miller E J (1974). Collagen polymorphism. Characterization of molecules with the chain composition $[1(III)]_3$ in human tissues. Science 183: 1200.

Chung E, Rhodes R K, Miller E J (1976). Isolation of three collagenous components of probable basement membrane origin from several tissues. Biochem Biophys Res Commun 71: 1167.

Claesson H E, Malmsten C (1977). On the interrelationship of prostaglandin endoperoxide G_2 and cyclic nucleotides in platelet function. Europ J Biochem 76: 277.

Fauvel F, Legrand Y J, Caen J P (1978). Platelet adhesion to type I collagen and $\alpha 1(I)_3$ trimers: Involvement of the C-terminal $\alpha 1(I)$ CB6A peptide. Thromb Res 12: 273.

Freytag J W, Dalrymple P N, Maguire M H, Strickland D K, Carraway K L, Hudson B G (1978). Glomerular basement membrane: Studies on its structure and interaction with platelets. J Biol Chem 253: 9069.

Furoto D K, Miller E J (1980). Isolation of a unique collagenous fraction from limited pepsin digests of human placental tissue. J. Biol Chem 255: 290.

Gastpar H, Kühn K, Marx R (eds) (1978). "Collagen-platelet interaction". New York: Schattauer.

Gay S, Balleisen L, Remberger K, Fietzek P P, Adelmann B C, Kühn K (1975). Immunohistochemical evidence for the presence of collagen type III in human arterial walls, arterial thrombi and in leucocytes, incubated with collagen in vitro. Klin Wochen 53: 899.

Gordon J L (ed) (1976). "Platelets in Biology and Pathology". Amsterdam: Elsevier/North Holland Biomedical Press.

Hovig T (1963). Aggregation of rabbit blood platelets produced in vitro by saline 'extract' of tendons. Thromb Diath Haem 9: 248.

Huang T W, Benditt E P (1978). Mechanism of platelet adhesion to the basal lamina. Am J Path 92: 99.

Huang T W, Lagunoff D, Benditt E P (1974). Nonaggregative adherence of platelets to basal lamina in vitro. Lab Invest 31: 156.

Hugues J (1960). Accolement des plaquettes au collagene. Comp Rend Seances Societe Biol, Paris 154: 866.

Hugues J, Herion F, Nusgens B, Lapiere C M (1976). Type III collagen and probably not type I collagen aggregates platelets. Throm Res 9: 223.

Jaffe R M (1976). Interaction of platelets with connective tissue. In Gordon J L (ed): "Platelets in Biology and Pathology". Amsterdam: Elsevier/North Holland Biomedical Press, p261.

Jaffe R M, Deykin D (1974). Evidence for a structural requirement for the aggregation of platelets by collagen. J Clin Invest 53: 875.

Kjaerheim A, Hovig T (1962). The ultrastructure of haemostatic blood platelet plugs in rabbit mesenterium. Thromb Diath Haem 7: 1.

Lages B, Weiss H J (1980). Biphasic aggregation responses to ADP and epineprine in some storage pool deficient platelets: relationship to the role of endogenous ADP in platelet aggregation and secretion. Thromb Haem 43: 147.

McCullagh K G, Balian G (1975). Collagen characterization cell transformation in human atherosclerosis. Nature, Lond 258: 73.

McCullagh K G, Duance V C, Bishop K A (1980). The distribution of collagen types I, III and V (AB) in normal and atherosclerotic human aorta. J Path 130: 45.

Moncada S, Amezcua J L (1979). Prostacyclin, thromboxane A_2 interactions in haemostasis and thrombosis. Haem 8: 252.

Moncada S, Vane J R (1978). Unstable metabolites of arachidonic acid and their role in haemostasis and thrombosis. In Thomas D (ed): "Thrombosis" Brit Med Bull 34: 129.

Muggli R, Baumgartner H R (1973). Collagen-induced platelet aggregation: requirement for tropocollagen multimers. Thromb Res 3: 715.

Mustard J F, Kinlough-Rathbone R L, Packham M A (1980). Prostaglandins and platelets. Ann Rev Med 31: 89.

Niewiarowski S, Stuart R K, Thomas D P (1966). Activation of intravascular coagulation by collagen. Proc Soc Exp Biol Med 123: 196.

Nordoy A (ed) (1979). "Blood vessel wall interactions in thrombogenesis". Haem 8: 121.

Nunn B (1979). Collagen-induced platelet aggregation: evidence against the essential role of platelet adenosine diphosphate. Thromb Haem 42: 1193.

Osterud B (1979). The role of endothelial cells and subendothelial components in the initiation of blood coagulation. Haem 8: 324.

Osterud B, Rapoport S I, Lavine K K (1977). Factor V activity of platelets: evidence for an activated factor V molecule and for a platelet activator. Blood 49: 819.

Ross R, Glomset J A (1976). The pathogenesis of atherosclerosis. New Eng J Med 295: 369,420.

Santoro S A, Cunningham L W (1977). Collagen-mediated platelet aggregation: evidence for multivalent interactions of intermediate specificity between collagen and platelets. J Clin Invest 60: 1054.

Thomas D (ed) (1977). "Haemostasis" Brit Med Bull 33: 183.

Thomas D (ed) (1978). "Thrombosis". Brit Med Bull 34: 101.

Trelstad R L (1974). Human aorta collagens: evidence for three distinct species. Biochem Biophys Res Commun 57: 717.

Trelstad R L, Carvalho A C A (1979). Type IV and type 'A-B' collagens do not elicit platelet aggregation or the serotonin release reaction. J Lab Clin Med 93: 499.

Trelstad R L, Lawley K R (1977). Isolation and initial characterization of human basement membrane collagens. Biochem Biophys Res Commun 76: 376.

Wall R T, Harker L A (1980). The endothelium and thrombosis. Ann Rev Med 31: 361.

Walsh P N (1972). The effects of collagen and kaolin on the intrinsic coagulation activities of platelets: evidence for an alternate pathway in intrinsic coagulation not requiring factor XII. Brit J Haematol 22: 393.

Wang C H, Miyata T, Weksler B, Rubin A L, Stenzel K H (1978). Collagen-induced platelet aggregation and release II. Critical size and structural requirements of collagen. Biochim Biophys Acta 544: 568.

Wharton-Jones T (1851). On the state of the blood and the blood vessels in inflammation. Guy's Hosp Rep 7: 1.

Wilner G D, Nossel H L, LeRoy E C (1968). Activation of Hageman factor by collagen. J Clin Invest 47: 2608.

Zacharski K R, Rosenstein R (1977). Further comments on the failure of collagen to activate factor XII. Thromb Res 10: 771.

Zucker M B (1980). The functioning of blood platelets. Scientific American 242: 70.

Zucker M B, Borelli J (1962). Platelet clumping produced by connective tissue suspensions and by collagen. Proc Soc Exp Biol Med 109: 779.

Connective Tissue Research:
Chemistry, Biology, and Physiology, Pages 183–194
© 1981 Alan R. Liss, Inc., 150 Fifth Avenue, New York, N.Y. 10011

THE MYOFIBROBLAST: A KEY CELL FOR WOUND HEALING AND
FIBROCONTRACTIVE DISEASES

Giulio GABBIANI

Department of Pathology, University of Geneva,
40 Boulevard de la Cluse, 1211 Geneva 4,
Switzerland.

Two phenomena play an essential role for the closing of
an open wound: one is formation and contraction of granulation tissue, and the second is epithelialization, i.e. movement and replication of epithelial cells over the wounded
area. Similarly to placenta during pregnancy, granulation
tissue is a new and temporary organ which disappears as soon
as the wound is closed by epithelialization. The main fonc-
tions of granulation tissue are: 1) synthesis of new connective tissue, and 2) production of a contractile movement
which brings together the margins of the wound. Old experiments by Carrel (1916) had shown that this contractile force
is produced within the granulation tissue itself. We have
studied the morphologic, functional and pharmacological characteristics of fibroblasts under normal conditions and
during wound healing or fibrocontractive diseases. Our
results indicate that during wound healing and fibrocontractive diseases, fibroblasts assume several characteristics of
smooth muscle cells. These modified fibroblasts or myofibroblasts probably play the key role in granulation tissue
contraction or in pathological connective tissue retractions.
We shall now review the characteristics of normal fibroblasts
and of myofibroblasts.

THE NORMAL FIBROBLAST

The fibroblast (Ross, 1968) was first identified by
means of light microscopy on the base of its shape and its

relationship with the extracellular substance. The use of
electron microscopy has allowed a better definition of the
cytological characteristics of fibroblasts. The nucleus is
generally large and contains one or more nucleoli. The most
prominent cytoplasmic organelle is rough endoplasmic reticulum which consists of a series of interconnected sack-like
or tubular structures present throughout the cytoplasm. The
content of these cisterns is relatively dense and sometimes
finely filamentous (Movat and Fernando, 1962; Ross and
Benditt, 1961); ribosomes form large aggregates on the membrane (Palade, 1958; Ross, 1968). The Golgi apparatus is
generally prominent and has no particular location (Ross,
1968). Abundant mitochondria are present throughout the
cytoplasm. Only a few cytoplasmic microfilaments (40-70 Å
in diameter) and intermediate filaments (100 Å in diameter)
may be seen in fibroblasts of adult animals or humans particularly close to the plasmalemma (Ross and Benditt, 1961).
In normal tissues of adult animals, there are no contacts
between fibroblasts. However, contacts can be seen between
embryonic and fetal fibroblasts as well as between fibroblasts of newborn animals (Greenle and Ross, 1967; Ross and
Greenle, 1966; Trelstad et al., 1970). These contacts most
commonly take the form of tight junctions.

THE MYOFIBROBLAST

In granulation tissue of normal wounds or in pathologic
connective tissue during fibrocontractive diseases (e.g.
Dupuytren's nodule), fibroblasts assume several new features.

Morphology

A fibrillar system develops within the cytoplasm
(Gabbiani et al., 1971); not the few fibrils seen in normal
fibroblasts, but bundles of parallel fibrils resembling those
of smooth muscle cells. Individual fibrils measure 40-80 Å
in diameter (more rarely 100-120 Å) and are usually arranged
parallel to the long axis of the cell. Many electron-opaque
areas are scattered among the bundles or located beneath the
plasmalemma. These are similar to the attachment sites of
smooth muscle. Although the fibrillar structures often
occupy a large portion of the cell, the remaining cytoplasm

contains packed cisterns of rough endoplasmic reticulum typical of normal fibroblasts. The nuclei show multiple indentations or deep folds, an appearance quite unlike that of
normal fibroblasts (or other cells in the same granulation
tissue such as macrophages or mast cells). There are numerous intercellular connections between granulation tissue
fibroblasts. Their structure identifies them as gap junctions (Gabbiani et al., 1978). In addition, part of the cell
surface is often covered by a well-defined layer of material
having the structural features of a basal lamina and generally separated from the cell membrane by a translucent layer.
Where it is covered by a basal lamina, the cell often shows
dense zones in the fibrillar bundles immediately beneath the
surface membrane. The resulting complex is reminiscent of
hemidesmosomes which bind endothelial cells, pericytes, and
smooth muscle cells to their basal laminae.

Pharmacology

    Strips of granulation tissue from animals or humans
placed in a pharmacological bath behave like smooth muscle
in that they are contracted or relaxed by substances that
contract or relax smooth muscle (Majno et al., 1971; Ryan
et al., 1973; Ryan et al., 1974). Among the substances most
active in inducing contraction are: 5-hydroxytriptamine
(5-HT or serotonin), angiotensin, vasopressin, norepinephri-
ne, bradykinin, epinephrine, and prostaglandin $F_{1\alpha}$.

Chemistry

    The yield of actomyosin obtained by extraction from a
croton oil-induced granuloma pouch (4.0 mg of actomyosin per
gram wet weight of pouch tissue) is comparable to that obtained with identically prepared extracts of pregnant rat
uteri (3.5 mg/g wet weight) (Majno et al., 1971). The
calcium-activated adenosine-triphosphatase activity of these
extracts is similar, splitting approximately 10 nM of adenosine triphosphate per mg or protein per min.

Immunology

Granulation tissue fibroblasts gradually develop intracellular neoantigens which are similar to those present in
smooth muscle cells. Thus, they fix anti-actin and antimyosin antibodies (Gabbiani et al., 1978). This gives
further support to the possibility that a mechanism involving
an interaction between actin and myosin is implicated in the
contraction of granulation tissue. When granulation tissue
disappears after the healing of a wound, no more fixation of
anti-actin and antimyosin antibodies to granulation tissue
fibroblasts is observed.

Collagen Synthesis

In inflamed tissues, collagen is synthesized more rapidly and is present in a higher concentration than in normal
tissues (Madden and Peacock, 1971). When the inflammatory
reaction subsides, collagen is progressively resorbed, and
the repaired tissue returns to normal composition. Collagen
from acutely or chronically inflamed tissue is less soluble
than collagen from normal tissue. This corresponds to the
presence in granulation tissue collagen of crosslinks different from those present in collagen of normal skin, but
similar to those present in collagen of embryonic skin
(Bailey et al., 1973; Hansen, 1975). Moreover, granulation
tissue induced in the rat by subcutaneous injection of tur-
pentine oil or by subcutaneous implantation of polyvinyl
sponges, contains a higher proportion of type III collagen
than normal skin (Bailey et al., 1975). Myofibroblasts are
present while the tissue is synthesizing type III collagen
and disappear when normal type I collagen with different
stabilizing crosslinks is being synthesized (Gabbiani et al,
1976). Therefore it appears probable that myofibroblasts
are, at least in part, responsible for the synthesis of
type III collagen. The collagen in normal skin is almost
totally of the classic type I, the fibers of which possess a
typical 640-Å periodicity, whereas in granulation tissue it
is composed of relatively few classic collagen fibers, some
fibers without periodicity, and a significant quantity of
finely filamentous material. It may be speculated that the
small filaments and the fibers without periodicity are

composed mainly of type III collagen. These fibers are probably analogous to those generally referred to as reticulin.
It is worth noting that type III collagen is present in tissues that need a certain plasticity, such as embryonic skin,
normal smooth muscle and granulation tissue. An increased
amount of type III collagen has been found in nodules of
Dupuytren's disease compared with normal palmar aponeurosis
(Bazin et al., 1980). Cultivated fibroblasts obtained from
chronically inflamed human gengiva produce increased amounts
of type III collagen when compared to fibroblasts obtained
from noninflamed tissues (Narayanan et al., 1978).

CONCLUSION

It is now widely accepted that the forces producing
wound contraction reside in the granulation tissue that fills
the wound. The nature of these forces however, has not been
clearly defined. The development of new features in fibroblasts of granulation tissue has led to the suggestion that
the characteristic contraction of granulation tissue depends
ultimately on the contraction of these modified fibroblasts
or myofibroblasts (Gabbiani et al., 1972) (Fig. 1). Fibroblasts cultivated in vitro develop an extensive cytoplasmic
fibrillar system, and interconnections in the form of gap
junctions. Contractile proteins can be isolated from these
cultivated cells (Adelstein et al., 1972; Bray and Thomas,
1975) or stained by means of immunofluorescence (Gabbiani et
al., 1973; Lazarides and Weber, 1974; Painter et al., 1975;
Weber and Groeschel-Stewart, 1974). In cultivated fibroblasts obtained from normal rat dermis, we observed that the
addition of 5-HT to the culture medium caused cellular con-
tractions within 15-20 min, whereas tryptophan had no effect
under the same conditions (Majno et al., 1971). The force
developed by a sheet of fibroblasts free from the substratum
in culture has been measured and has been found to be about
the same per unit cross-sectional area as that of granulation
tissue of a wound and about 1/10 of that of smooth muscle
(James and Taylor, 1969).

Myofibroblasts have been described in man and animals
during several pathologic situations. Some of these situations are inflammatory in nature and related to wound healing
(Ariyan et al., 1978; Baur et al., 1975; Baur et al., 1977;

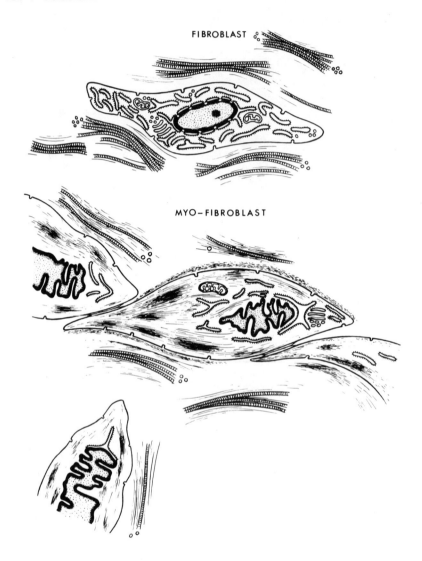

FIBROBLAST

MYO–FIBROBLAST

Figure 1.- Scheme comparing the characteristics of fibroblasts. The upper part of the figure shows a typical fibroblast with a smooth contour of the nucleus which contains a
nucleolus. The cytoplasm contains cisternae of rough endoplasmic reticulum, mitochondria, a Golgi apparatus, and pe-
ripheral vesicles, but only few intracytoplasmic fibrils.

The lower part of the figure shows an area of granulation
tissue. The cellular concentration is higher than in normal
connective tissue. Myofibroblasts have a nucleus with numerous folds and indentations. The cytoplasm still has some
cisternae of rough endoplasmic reticulum, but its most characteristic feature is the presence of massive bundles of filaments usually arranged parallel to the long axis of the cell.
Electron-dense areas are scattered among the bundles or located beneath the plasmalemma. Intercellular connections in
the form of gap junctions are present between fibroblasts.
In addition, a part of the cell surface is often covered by
a well-defined layer of material similar to a basal lamina.
In such regions, the cell commonly shows a dense zone (giving
a hemidesmosome complex) in the fibrillar bundles immediately
beneath the surface membrane (from Gabbiani et al., 1973 and
from Gabbiani [1979] Meth Achiev exp Pathol 9:187).

Dabelsteen and Kremenak, 1978; Grimaud and Borojevic, 1977;
Guber and Rudolph, 1978; Larson et al., 1974; Madden, 1973;
Peacock, 1978; Roland, 1976; Rudolph and Woodward, 1978;
Rudolph et al., 1977; Rudolph et al., 1978; Zimman et al.,
1978). Some are connected to the so-called fibromatoses
(Benjamin et al., 1977; Chiu et al., 1978; Feiner and Kaye,
1976; Fisher et al., 1978; Gabbiani and Majno, 1972; Gokel
and Hübner, 1977; Hueston et al., 1976; Katenkamp and Stiller,
1975; Madden et al., 1975; Schwarzlmüller and Hofstädter,
1978; Weathers and Campbell, 1974; Wirman, 1976) and in some
cases the pathogenesis is unknown, e.g. liver cirrhosis
(Bhathal, 1972; Rudolph et al., 1979) or kidney fibrosis
(Nagle et al., 1975). Finally, there are few reports of
malignant myofibroblastic tumors (Churg and Kahn, 1977;
Stiller and Katenkamp, 1975; Vasudev and Harris, 1978;
d'Andiran and Gabbiani, in press).

It appears that in experimental animals or humans, the
fibroblast is a very plastic cell which can adapt to different situations by changing morphological, biochemical and
functional features. Thus, during wound healing there is a
transformation of local fibroblasts and/or other less differentiated cells into myofibroblasts (Gabbiani et al., 1972).
These acquire many properties typical of cultivated fibroblasts and in particular an important contractile apparatus

which is probably responsible for the mechanism of granulation tissue contraction.

A relationship between intracytoplasmic filaments and cellular motion, development of tension, and intracytoplasmic movements or secretion has been proposed for a wide spectrum of cells ranging from monocellular organisms to those of mammalian tissues (Pollard and Weihing, 1974). The development of a contractile filamentous apparatus probably takes place when cells of different embryological origin face situations that require the enhancement of certain characteristic functions, such as the ability to move about and to contract. In granulation tissue, the contraction of a single myofibroblast is then transmitted to other cells and to the stroma; this response is synchronized rather than individual.

Acknowledgements. We thank Academic Press, London and S. Karger, Basel, for granting the permission of reproducing Figure 1. Supported in part by the Swiss National Science Foundation, Grant Nr 3.445-0.79.

REFERENCES

Adelstein RS, Conti MA, Johnson GS, Pastan I (1972). Isolation and characterization of myosin from cloned mouse fibroblasts. Proc Natl Acad Sci USA 69:3693.
Ariyan S, Enriquez R, Krizek TJ (1978). Wound contraction and fibrocontractive disorders. Arch Surg 113:1034.
Bailey AJ, Bazin S, Delaunay A (1973). Changes in the nature of the collagen during development and resorption of granulation tissue. Biochim Biophys Acta 328:383.
Bailey AJ, Sims TJ, Le Lous M, Bazin S (1975). Collagen polymorphism in experimental granulation tissue. Biochem Biophys Res Commun 66:1160.
Baur PS, Larson DL, Stacey TR (1975). The observation of myofibroblasts in hypertrophic scars. Surg Gynecol Obstet 141:22.
Baur PS, Parks DH, Larson DL (1977). The healing of burn wounds. Clin Plast Surg 4:389.
Bazin S, Le Lous M, Duance VC, Sims TJ, Bailey AJ, Gabbiani G, d'Andiran G, Pizzolato G, Browski A, Nicoletis C, Delaunay A (1980). Biochemistry and histology of the connective tissue of Dupuytren's disease lesions. Eur J Clin Invest 10:9.

Benjamin SP, Mercer RD, Hawk WA (1977). Myofibroblastic contraction in spontaneous regression of multiple congenital mesenchymal hamartomas. Cancer 40:2343.

Bhathal PS (1972). Presence of modified fibroblasts in cirrhotic livers in man. Pathology 4:139.

Bray D, Thomas C (1975). The actin consert of fibroblasts. Biochem J 147:221.

Carrel A (1916). Cicatrisation of wounds. I. The relation between the size of a wound and the rate of its cicatrisation. J Exp Med 24:429.

Chiu HF, McFarlane RM (1978). Pathogenesis of Dupuytren's contracture: a correlative clinical-pathological study. J Hand Surg 3:1.

Churg AM, Kahn LB (1977). Myofibroblasts and related cells in malignant fibrous and fibrohistiocytic tumors. Hum Pathol 8:205.

Dabelsteen E, Kremenak CR (1978). Demonstration of actin in the fibroblasts of healing palatal wounds. Plast Reconstr Surg 62:429.

D'Andiran G, Gabbiani G (in press). A metastasizing sarcoma of the pleura composed of myofibroblasts. In Fenoglio CM, Wolff M (eds): "Progress in Surgical Pathology, Vol II," New York: Masson.

Feiner H, Kaye GI (1976). Ultrastructural evidence of myofibroblasts in circumscribed fibromatosis. Arch Pathol Lab Med 100:265.

Fisher ER, Paulson JD, Gregorio RM (1978). The myofibroblastic nature of the uterine plexiform tumor. Arch Pathol Lab Med 102:477.

Gabbiani G, Majno G (1972). Dupuytren's contracture: fibroblast contraction? An ultrastructural study. Am J Pathol 66:131.

Gabbiani G, Ryan GB, Majno G (1971). Presence of modified fibroblasts in granulation tissue and their possible role in wound contraction. Experientia 27:549.

Gabbiani G, Hirschel BJ, Ryan GB, Statkov PR, Majno G (1972). Granulation tissue as a contractile organ. A study of structure and function. J Exp Med 135:719.

Gabbiani G, Majno G, Ryan GB (1973). The fibroblast as a contractile cell: the myofibroblast. In Kulonen E, Pikkarainen J (eds): "Biology of Fibroblast," London: Academic Press, p 139.

Gabbiani G, Le Lous M, Bailey AJ, Bazin S, Delaunay A (1976) Collagen and myofibroblasts of granulation tissue. A chemical, ultrastructural and immunologic study. Virchows Arch [Cell Pathol] 21:133.

Gabbiani G, Chaponnier C, Hüttner I (1978). Cytoplasmic filaments and gap junctions in epithelial cells and myofibroblasts during wound healing. J Cell Biol 76:561.

Gokel JM, Hübner G (1977). Occurrence of myofibroblasts in the different phases of morbus Dupuytren (Dupuytren's contracture). Beitr Pathol 161:166.

Greenle TK, Ross R (1967). The development of the rat flexor digital tendon. A fine structure study. J Ultrastruct Res 18:354.

Grimaud JA, Borojevic R (1977). Myofibroblasts in hepatic schistosomal fibrosis. Experientia 33:890.

Guber S, Rudolph R (1978). The myofibroblast. Surg Gynecol Obstet 146:641.

Hansen TM (1975). Collagen development in granulation tissue as compared with collagen of skin and aorta from injured and non-injured rats. Acta Pathol Microbiol Scand [A] 83:721.

Hueston JT, Hurley VJ, Whittingham S (1976). The contracting fibroblast as a clue to Dupuytren's contracture. The Hand 8:10.

James DW, Taylor JF (1969). The stress developed by sheets of chick fibroblasts in vitro. Exp Cell Res 54:107.

Katenkamp D, Stiller D (1975). Cellular composition of the so-called dermatofibroma (histiocytoma cutis). Virchows Arch [Pathol Anat] 367:325.

Larson DL, Abston S, Willis B, Linares H, Dobrkovsky M, Evans EB, Lewis SR (1974). Contracture and scar formation in the burn patient. Clin Plast Surg 1:653.

Lazarides E, Weber K (1974). Actin antibody: the specific visualization of actin filaments in non-muscle cells. Proc Natl Acad Sci USA 71:2268.

Madden JW (1973). On "the contractile fibroblast". Plast Reconstr Surg 52:291.

Madden JW, Peacock EE (1971). Studies on the biology of collagen during wound healing. III. Dynamic metabolism of scar collagen and remodeling of dermal wounds. Ann Surg 174:511.

Madden JW, Carlson EC, Hines J (1975). Presence of modified fibroblasts in ischemic contracture of the intrinsic musculature of the hand. Surg Gynecol Obstet 140:509.

Majno G, Gabbiani G, Hirschel BJ, Ryan GB, Statkov PR (1971).
Contraction of granulation tissue in vitro: similarity to
smooth muscle. Science 173:548.

Movat HZ, Fernando NVP (1962). The fine structure of connective tissue. I. The fibroblast. Exp Mol Pathol 1:509.

Nagle RB, Evans LW, Reynolds DG (1975). Contractility of
renal cortex following complete ureteral obstruction. Proc
Soc exp Biol Med 148:611.

Narayanan AS, Page RC, Kuzan F (1978). Collagens synthesized
in vitro by diploid fibroblasts obtained from chronically
inflamed human connective tissue. Lab Invest 39:61.

Painter RG, Sheetz M, Singer SJ (1975). Detection and ultrastructural localization of human smooth muscle myosin-like
molecules in human nonmuscle cells by specific antibodies.
Proc Natl Acad Sci USA 72:1359.

Palade (1958). A small particulate component of the cytoplasm.
In Sandford LP (ed): "Frontiers in Cytology," New Haven:
Yale University Press, p 283.

Peacock EE (1978). Wound contraction and scar contracture.
Plast Reconstr Surg 62:600.

Pollard TD, Weihing RR (1974). Actin and myosin and cell movement. In Fassman GD (ed): "CRC Critical Review of Biochemistry, Vol 2," Cleveland: Chemical Rubber Company, p 1.

Roland J (1976). Fibroblaste et myofibroblaste dans le pro-
cessus granulomateux. Ann Anat Pathol 21:37.

Ross R (1968). The connective tissue fiber forming cell. In
Ramachandran GN (ed): "Treatise on Collagen, Vol 2, Part
A," New York: Academic Press, p 1.

Ross R, Benditt EP (1961). Wound healing and collagen formation. I. Sequential changes in components of guinea pig
skin wounds observed in the electron microscope. J Biophys
Biochem Cytol 11:677.

Ross R, Greenle TK (1966). Electron microscopy: attachment
sites between connective tissue cells. Science 153:997.

Rudolph R, Woodward M (1978). Spatial orientation of microtubules in contractile fibroblasts in vivo. Anat Rec 191:
169.

Rudolph R, Guber S, Suzuki M, Woodward M (1977). The life
cycle of the myofibroblast. Surg Gynecol Obstet 145:389.

Rudolph R, Abraham J, Vecchione T, Guber S, Woodward M (1978).
Myofibroblasts and free silicon around breast implants.
Plast Reconstr Surg 62:185.

Rudolph R, McClure WJ, Woodward M (1979). Contractile fibroblasts in chronic alcoholic cirrhosis. Gastroenterol 76:704.

Ryan GB, Cliff WJ, Gabbiani G, Irle C, Statkov PR, Majno G (1973). Myofibroblasts in an avascular fibrous tissue. Lab Invest 29:197.

Ryan GB, Cliff WJ, Gabbiani G, Irle C, Montandon D, Statkov PR, Majno G (1974). Myofibroblasts in human granulation tissue. Hum Pathol 5:55.

Schwarzlmüller B, Hofstädter F (1978). Fibromatose der Schilddrüsenregion. Eine elektronenmikroskopische und enzymhistochemische Studie. Virchows Arch [Pathol Anat] 377:145.

Stiller D, Katenkamp D (1975). Cellular features in desmoid fibromatosis and well-differentiated fibrosarcomas. An electron microscopic study. Virchows Arch [Pathol Anat] 369:155.

Trelstad RL, Kang AH, Igarashi S, Gross J (1970). Isolation of two distinct collagens from chick cartilage. Biochemistry 9:4993.

Vasudev KS, Harris M (1978). A sarcoma of myofibroblasts. An ultrastructural study. Arch Pathol Lab Med 102:185.

Weathers DR, Campbell WG (1974). Ultrastructure of the giant-cell fibroma of the oral mucosa. Oral Surg 38:550.

Weber K, Groeschel-Stewart U (1974). Antibody to myosin: the specific visualization of myosin-containing filaments in nonmuscle cells. Proc Natl Acad Sci USA 71:4561.

Wirman JA (1976). Nodular fasciitis, a lesion of myofibroblasts. An ultrastructural study. Cancer 38:2378.

Zimman OA, Robles JM, Lee JC (1978). The fibrous capsule around mammary implants: an investigation. Aest Plast Surg 2:217.

Connective Tissue Research:
Chemistry, Biology, and Physiology, Pages 195–207
© 1981 Alan R. Liss, Inc., 150 Fifth Avenue, New York, N.Y. 10011

BEHAVIOUR OF COLLAGEN IN DIFFERENT HUMAN DISEASES

M. Adam, Z. Deyl and L. Miterová

Res. Inst. Rheum. Diseases and
Inst. of Physiology, Czech. Acad. Sci.,
Prague, Czechoslovakia.

With the development of molecular biology a new era of pathology was started. Many physiological pathways were elucidated on the molecular level and it was possible, therefore, to look after pathological alterations on the same level. Literature provides a basis for initiating a classification of diseases from the molecular point of view and for explaining of various clinical symptoms with structural or metabolic disturbances of respective substances.

Collagen, actually collagens, since there is a closely related family of proteins with similar structure, is one of the most important component of connective tissue. Collagens are the most abundant of mammalian proteins, being distributed throughout the body. They form a scaffold on which structures such as the cornea are built. Providing strength and integrity collagen serves principally as a structural component in organs that bear weight, transmit force or light, protect or compartmentalize, and distribute fluids. The functions of collagen are, however, more diverse: it affects body hemostasis through interaction with platelets and it is an important component of basement membranes. Further, collagen determines whether processes such as metamorphosis and organogenesis, tissue remodelling and wound healing will follow a normal or pathological course. It has been demonstrated, that collagen is essential for the epithelial - epithelial and epithelial - mesenchymal interactions and plays an important role in cell differentiation. While the growth and differentiation promoting effect of collagen is associated with its precisely timed synthesis, the production of abnormal collagen type brings about alteration in tissue formation and metabolism. Thus, it is now evident that collagen is not only the major structural protein which functions via its fibers to stabilize the body organs, but even it is essential for cytodifferentiation. Therefore, all alterations in its structure or metabolism may further affect cell function. On the other hand it is known that changes in the environment of cells may result in a change in the types of collagen being synthesized.

Collagen is involved in a wide variety of disorders. The ultimate resistance of collagen polymers to stress and the organization of the molecules in the fibers are closely related to the structure of the collagen monomer. Malfunction of any step in collagen metabolism may therefore lead to its defective properties - mechanical, transportive, depository etc.

No precise information is available about control in the use of the different collagen cistrons. Some disease could be attributed to an abnormal expression of the genetic information. Some others are caused by defects of some processes participating in posttranslational collagen modifications or in blocking these modifications by another mechanism. From what was said it is apparent that alterations in collagen metabolism or structure may cause a broad variety of clinical symptoms.

Since the primary functions of collagen are to determine the tensile strength and extensibility of tissues, it is not surprising that tissue fragility and/or hyperextensibility are features of the many heritable disorders of collagen. These disorders include the Ehlers-Danlos syndromes, which are linked historically, but we know now that they vary clinically, genetically and biochemically (Lichtenstein et al., 1973; Pope et al., 1975). Each group can be defined by a subset of distinct clinical findings and in some cases by a defined biochemical lesion (Tab. 1). The inborn errors of collagen metabolism include further some specific entities that are classified as osteogenesis imperfecta (Penttinen et al., 1975), the Marfan syndrome (Siegel and Chang, 1978) cutis laxa (Byers et al., 1976). Menkes' kinky hair syndrome (Danks and Cartwright, 1973). There is also at least one heritable disease, homocystinuria (Kang and Trelstand, 1973), in which the metabolism of collagen is secondary affected.

TABLE 1

Inborn errors of collagen metabolism

Affected step in collagen metabolism	Manifestations designed as:
Regulation of synthesis	Osteogenesis imperfecta Ehlers-Danlos syndrome type IV
Regulation of catabolism Collagenase	Epidermolysis bullosa

Posttranslational modifications of collagen
  Lysyl hydroxylase
  Glycosyl transferase
  Lysyl oxidase, Cu^{++}
	Ehlers-Danlos syndrome type VI
	Osteogenesis imperfecta
	Cutis laxa
	Marfan syndrome
	Menkes' kinky hair syndrome
	Homocystinuria
	Ochronosis

Transport effects and molecular packing Molecular packing	Ehlers-Danlos syndrome type I Spondyloepiphyseal dysplasia Mucopolysaccharidoses
Procollagen secretion Procollagen protease	Ehlers-Danlos syndrome type IV Ehlers-Danlos syndrome type VII

Most disease processes involve tissue injury, and the response to this injury very quickly results in a localized response of fibroblasts or mesenchymal cells. This localized response contrasts with the more generalized regulatory defects in heritable disorders of collagen and it includes usually a stimulation of both cell proliferation and extracellular matrix synthesis. The response to nearly all forms of tissue injury involves regulatory changes in the rates and/or the types of collagen synthesis (Tab. 2).

Changes in the amounts of collagen in the acquired diseases and repair processes are most apparent. An excess of collagen synthesis is a major problem mainly in parenchymatous organs. The amount of collagen synthesis is usually reflected by an increase in reducible cross-links in the tissues (Bailey et al., 1974). On the other hand acquired deficiences or blocks in the formation of cross-links or defects in the conversion of reducible cross-links to non-reducible ones are known. A decrease in the rate of conversion may result in an accumulation of reducible cross-links, while an increase in the rate of conversion may decrease the rate of degradation or turnover of collagen. Thus an increase in the conversion of cross-links may contribute to the development of fibrotic processes. It should be mentioned here that penicillamine used in the therapy of different diseases may block the formation of polyfunctional cross-links from the Schiff base cross-link precursor (Deshmukh and Nimni, 1969; Siegel, 1977).

In the early stages of fibrous tissue repair there is an increase in the synthesis of type III collagen (Gabbiani et al., 1976). As this repair progresses, there is a return to a marked predominance of type I collagen. Type III collagen is found in higher concentrations in early scar tissue than in surrounding dermis (Craig et al., 1975; Barnes et al., 1975; Shuttleworth et al., 1975). The high proportion of type III collagen persists in pathological scars long after the collagen type pattern in normal scars has reverted to that seen in normal dermis. Biochemical studies of Dupuytren's disease, contractures and nodules have revealed an increase in type III collagen and in reducible aldimine cross-links (Bailey et al., 1977).

It is likely that enhanced type III collagen synthesis and deposition will be found in a variety of inflammatory

TABLE 2

Changes of collagen metabolism in some acquired diseases and repair processes

Disorder	Increase of the biosynthesis	Increase of some collagen type	Increase in the cross-links concetration	Break-down
Dupuytren's contracture		+		
Osteoarthrosis	+	+		increased
Rheumatoid arthritis	+	+		increased
Pulmonary fibrosis	+	+		
Liver cirrhosis	+	+	+	
Atherosclerosis	+	+		
Neoplasia	+	+	+ (?)	+
Diabetes mellitus	+			
Hypertrophic scar	+	+	+	
Scleroderma	+	+	+	decreased
Osteopetrosis	+		+	decreased

states and in response to diverse injuries as has been reported in rheumatoid arthritis, scleroderma, bronchopneumonia, experimental granuloma etc. (Tab. 3) (Adam et al., (1979).

Fibrotic states are associated with excessive synthesis and deposition of collagen, in a manner that distorts the normal architecture and compromises the function of the organ. In pulmonary fibrosis the relative content of type III collagen is markedly diminished and the degree of hydroxylation of lysyl residues is reduced (Crystal et al., 1976; Hance and Crystal, 1975; Seyer et al., 1976). Immunofluorescent studies have confirmed the marked increase in types I and V collagen, while type III collagen was found to be reduced in alveolar septae. The increase in the proportion of type I collagen leads to a more rigid, less distensible tissue with reduced compliance (Madri and Furthmayr, 1979). Several reports indicate that both a relative and an absolute increase in type III collagen in the interlobular spaces of liver in the acute response to injury (Gay et al., 1975; Rojkind et al., 1976). There is however a marked increase in type I collagen synthesis when the liver injury becomes irreversible (Seyer et al., 1977). Some alterations of collagen synthesis and deposition occurs also in atheromatous arterial walls - it seems that mainly synthesis of collagen type V is enhanced (Bečvář et al., 1980) and in plaque collagen type I may be increased (Mc Cullagh and Balian, 1975).

Human hyaline cartilage was reported to contain collagen type II only (Miller and Matukas, 1969). Indeed Nimni and Deshmukh (1973) showed that collagen with characteristics of type I was present in osteoarthritic cartilage. Studies of Adam et al. (to be published) have shown that also type III collagen is present in hyaline cartilage. Both collagen types I and III were found to be localized selectively in the pericellular region of chondrocytes (Fig. 1 a, b). Because both collagen types I and III were found also in the articular cartilage of persons in the third life decade without any clinical symptoms of osteoarthrosis it is rather difficult to decide at the moment if the presence of collagens type I and III is indicative for aging process or osteoarthrosis only. Simultaneously with the presence of collagen types I and III in osteoarthrotic cartilage the diminished collagen resistence against proteolytic digestion could be observed (Adam et al. 1976). It should be emphasized that also an-

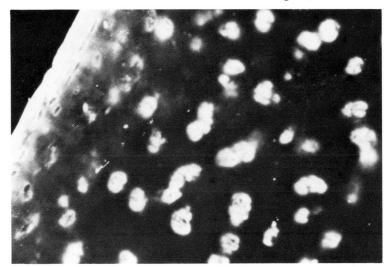

Fig. 1A. Human osteoarthrotic cartilage. Frozen sections
stained with anti-type I collagen antibodies. In the deeper
lacunal spaces multicellular clusters of chondrocytes are
surrounded with collagen type I.

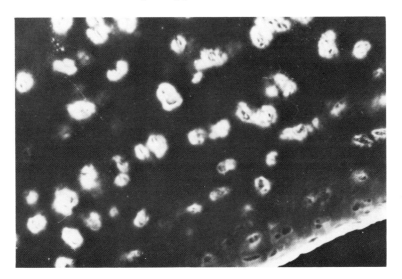

Fig. 1B. Human osteoarthrotic cartilage. Frozen sections
stained with anti-type III collagen antibodies. In the
deeper lacunal spaces multicellular clusters of chondrocytes
are surrounded with collagen type III, similarly as Fig. 1A,
where collagen type I is present.

TABLE 3

Collagen type III content from insoluble pepsin treated collagen in various tissues (in mg/g of total solubilized collagen) (Adam et al., 1979)

Investigated tissue	Normal			Diseased	
	46	53	62 years old		
Skin	221	208	191	SSM*	411
				Systemic scleroderma (48 years old)	362
Oesophagus	342	332	331	SSM	444
Heart muscle	325	337	301	SSM	408
Liver	391	379	382	SSM	458
				Cirrhosis, late stage (62 years old)	302
Lung	302	288	294	SSM	418
				Bronchopneumonia, 1st case (68 years old)	467
				2nd case (54 years old)	380
Kidney	351	340	312	SSM	430
Synovial tissue-24 years old	204			Rheumatoid arthritis (35 years old)	318
				Rheumatoid nodule (44 years old)	438

* SSM – Systemic scleroderma malignant (42 years old).

nulus fibrosus of intervertebral disc of adult persons contained besides collagen type II and I (Eyre and Muir, 1974) also type III collagen (Fig. 2 a, b) (Adam et al., to be published). We were able to determine the presence of collagen type III in osteoarthrotic cartilage also by biochemical methods. Our preliminary results indicate that the occurence of collagens type I and III in hyaline cartilage is accompanied with the presence of fibronectin, what may be in a relationship to the switch of collagen synthesis from type II to type I and III.

Cartilage is further altered in ochronosis, what is an inherited disorder of amino acid metabolism in which homogentisic acid and its oxidation products accumulate in tissues. Homogentisic acid or its oxidation product - benzoquinone acetic acid, may bind to a number of amino acids and also to collagen (Milch, 1962). The inhibition of lysyl hydroxylase by homogentisic acid was shown in recent studies that demonstrated the reduction of the number of hydroxylysine-derived cross-links (Murray et al. 1977). The products of homogentisic acid reactions could therefore alter collagen in vivo and thus contribute to the development of ochronotic arthropathy.

Also spondyloepiphyseal dysplasia appears to be caused by an abnormality in the formation or stability of fibrils in various tissues (Byers et al. 1978).

Several disorders appear to be associated with abnormalities of collagenase sometimes determined genetically. E.g. increased concentrations of collagenase are found in dermis of persons with epidermolysis bullosa (Bauer et al., 1977). The increased concentration of collagenase was found also in synovial fluid of patients with rheumatoid arthritis, in periodontal disease, corneal ulceration etc. On the other hand skin of patients with scleroderma is reported to contain low level concentrations of collagenase (Brady, 1975).

In conclusion, there is a number of known factors affecting collagen synthesis and the cell morphology. Further studies may contribute to elucidation of disorders such as atherosclerosis, the fibrotic diseases and may lead some day to a therapeutic regulation of collagen metabolism in tissues.

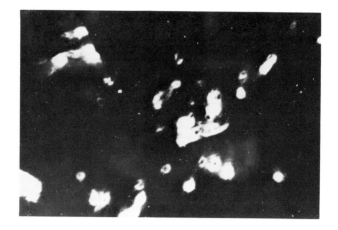

Fig. 2A. The annunulus fibrosus of human degenerated intervertebral disc. Frozen section stained with anti-type I
collagen antibodies. Multicellular clusters of cells are
surrounded with collagen staining positively for collagen
type I.

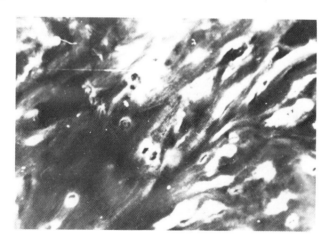

Fig. 2B. The annunulus fibrosus of human degenerated intervertebral disc. Frozen section stained with anti-type III
collagen antibodies. Multicellular clusters of cells are
surrounded with collagen staining positively for collagen
type III. Also some collagen fibers are positively stained.

REFERENCES

Adam M, Dostál C and Deyl Z (1979). Collagen heterogeneity in systemic scleroderma and other diseases. J Clin Chem Clin Biochem 17:495.

Adam M, Musilová J and Deyl Z (1976). Cartilage collagen in osteoarthrosis. Clin Chim Acta 69:53.

Bailey AJ, Robbins SP and Balian G (1974). Biological significance of the intermolecular crosslinks of collagen. Nature 25:105.

Bailey AJ, Sims TJ, Gabbiani G, Bazin S and Le Lous M (1977). Collagen of Dupuytren's disease. Clin Sci Mol Med 53:499.

Barnes MJ, Morton LF, Bailey AJ and Bennett RC (1975). Studies on collagen synthesis in the nature dermal scar in the guinea pig. Br Biochem Soc Trans 3:917.

Bauer EA, Gedde-Dahl T Jr and Eisen AE (1977). The role of human skin collagenase in epidermolysis bullosa. J Invest Derm 68:119.

Bečvář R, Miterová L and Adam M. Heterogeneity of collagen in atheromatous aorta. In "Abstract of VII. European Symposium on Connective Tissue Research", 8-11th September 1980, Prague.

Brady AH (1975). Collagenase in scleroderma. J Clin Invest 56:1175.

Byers PH, Holbrock KA, Hall JG, Bornstein P and Chandler JW (1978). A new variety of spondyloepiplyseal dysplasia characterized by punctate. Corneal dystrophy and abnormal dermal collagen fibrils. Human Genet 40:157.

Byers PH, Narayanan AS, Bornstein P and Hall JG (1976). An X-linked form of cutis laxa due to deficiency of lysyl oxidase. Birth Defects 12:293.

Craig RDP, Schofield JD and Jackson SS (1975). Collagen biosynthesis in normal human skin, normal and hypertrophic scar and keloid. Eur J Clin Invest 5:69.

Crystal RG, Fulmer JD, Roberts WC, Mors ML, Line BR and Reynolds HY (1976). Idiopathic pulmonary fibrosis: Clinical, histologic, radiographic, physiologic, scientigraphic, cytologic and histochemical aspects. Am Int Med 85:769.

Danks DM and Cartwright E (1973). Menkes' kinky hair disease: further definition of the defect in copper transport. Science 179:1140.

Deshmukh K and Nimni ME (1969). A defect in the intramolecular and intermolecular cross-linking of collagen caused by penicillamine. II. Functional groups involved in the interaction process. J Biol Chem 244:1787.

Eyre DR and Muir H (1974). Collagen polymorphism: two molecular species in pig intervertebral disc. FEBS Lett 42:192.

Gabbiani S, Le Lous M, Bailey AJ, Bazin S and Delaunay A (1976). Collagen and myofibroblasts of granulation tissue. A chemical, ultrastructural and immunologic study. Virchows Archiv (Cell Pathol) 21:133.

Gay S, Fietzek PP, Remberger K, Eder M and Kühn K (1975). Liver cirrhosis: Immunofluorescence and biochemical studies demonstrate two types of collagen. Klin Wschs 53:205.

Hance AJ and Crystal RG (1975). The connective tissue of lung. Am Rev Respir Dis 112:657.

Kang AH and Trelstand RL (1973). A collagen defect in homocystinuria. J Clin Invest 52:2571.

Lichtenstein JR, Martin GR, Kohn LD, Byers PH and Mc Kusick VA (1973). Defect in conversion of procollagen to collagen in a form of Ehlers-Danlos syndrome. Science 182:298.

Madri JA and Furthmayr H (1979). Isolation and tissue localization of type AB_2 collagen from lung parenchyma. AM J Pathol 94:323.

Mc Cullagh KA and Balian G (1975). Collagen characterization and cell transformation in human atherosclerosis. Nature 258:73.

Milch RA (1962). Biochemical studies on the pathogenesis of collagen tissue changes in alcaptonuria. Clin Orthoped 24:213.

Miller EJ and Matukas VY (1969). Chick cartilage collagen: A new type of α_1 chain not present in bone or skin of the species (1969). Proc Nat Acad Sci USA 64:1264.

Murray DC, Lindberg KA and Pinnell SR (1977). In vitro inhibition of chick embryo lysyl hydroxylase by homogentisic acid. J Clin Invest 59:1071.

Nimni M and Deshmukh K (1973). Differences in collagen metabolism between normal and osteoarthrotic human articular cartilage. Science 181:751.

Penttinen RP, Lichtenstein JR, Martin GR and McKusick VA (1975). Abnormal collagen metabolism in cultured cell in osteogenesis imperfecta. Proc Nat Acad Sci USA 72:586.

Pope FM, Martin GR, Lichtenstein JR, Penttinen R, Gerson B, Rowe DW and McKusick VA (1975). Patients with Ehlers-Danlose syndrome lack type III collagen. Proc Nat Acad Sci USA 72:1314.

Rojkind M and Martinez-Paloma A (1976). Increase in type I and type III collagens in human alcoholic liver cirrhosis. Proc Nat Acad Sci USA 73:539.

Seyer JM, Hutcheson ET and Kang AH (1976). Collagen polymorphism in idiopathic chronic pulmonary fibrosis. J Clin Invest 57:1498.

Seyer JM, Hutcheson ET and Kang AH (1977). Collagen polymorphism in normal and cirrhotic human liver. J Clin Invest 59:241.

Shuttleworth CA, Forrest L and Jackson DS (1975). Comparison of the cyanogen bromide peptides of insoluble guinea pig skin and scar collagen. Biochem Biophys Acta 379:207.

Siegel RC (1977). Collagen cross-linking: Effect of D-penicillamine on cross-linking in vitro. J Biol Chem 252:254.

Siegel RC and Chang YH (1978). Detective α_2 chain synthesis in patients with sporadic Marfan syndrome. Clin Res 26:501.

Connective Tissue Research:
Chemistry, Biology, and Physiology, Pages 209–218
© **1981 Alan R. Liss, Inc., 150 Fifth Avenue, New York, N.Y. 10011**

PHARMACOLOGICAL CONTROL OF INFLAMMATORY CONNECTIVE TISSUE
DISEASES

Ib Lorenzen

Hvidovre hospital
Department of Rheumatology
University of Copenhagen
Denmark

The inflammatory connective tissue diseases, i.e. inflammatory rheumatic diseases represent some of the most common
diseases. They are usually chronic diseases, and important
causes of disability. The major disease in this group is
rheumatoid arthritis. Other examples are the reactive or
postinfectious arthritides, systemic lupus erythematosus
and systemic vasculitis, among these giant cell arteritis
and polyarteritis nodosa.

The primary etiological factor and the early pathogenetic mechanisms are generally unknown. In all probability
the primary cause of the more important diseases is a microbial infection of bacterial or viral nature. Classical examples are rheumatic fever and other postinfectious arthritides. Possibly infection also play a role in the pathogenesis of rheumatoid arthritis and systemic lupus erythematosus, as well as in several types of systemic vasculitides.

However, a condition to the development of inflammatory rheumatic disease following microbial infection seems to
be an increased individual susceptibility to the primary microbial agent. The increased susceptibility may be due to an
alteration in the immune system or in the non specific mesenchymal reaction of inflammation and repair or both. The demonstration of the association between certain HLA-antigens
and some of the inflammatory rheumatic diseases suggest that
a defect in the immune system may be of importance.

The alterations in the immune system may imply a persistence of the primary microbial antigen and immunological hyperreactivity including autoimmune phenomena and secondary to this, a non specific process of inflammation and repair.

In contrast to the hypothetical microbial and immunological pathogenetic mechanisms inflammation is of inquestionable pathogenetic importance to the clinical symptoms in the inflammatory connective tissue disorders. Major evidence indicate that we are dealing with non specific processes of injury and repair. The explanation of the presence and persistence of inflammation will probably be found in the microbial and immunological reactions preceding and eliciting inflammation.

Our present knowledge on the etiology and pathogenesis of the inflammatory rheumatic diseases implies that the basis for the pharmacological therapy is a pharmacological control of the process of inflammation and repair in the connective tissue i.e. anti-inflammatory therapy.

The object of the anti-inflammatory therapy is <u>arthritis</u> with inflammation of joint capsule and joint cartilage and bone and different types of <u>extra-articular inflammation</u>. The extra-articular manifestations may be located to the vessel wall, <u>vasculitis</u> or more diffusely in the connective tissue, e.g. skin and muscels.

I shall mention some of the fundamental problems in the pharmacological control of the connective tissue reactions in the inflammatory connective tissue disorders:

a: Which type of drugs are at present the most promising drugs?
b: What is our present knowledge on their mechanism of action on the connective tissue?
c: Future trends and perspectives in pharmacological control of connective tissue reactions in inflammatory connective tissue disease?

ANTI-INFLAMMATORY DRUGS

The anti-inflammatory drugs in clinical use are the non-steroidal anti-inflammatory drugs and a group of stronger acting antirheumatic drugs, including antimarials, gold salts, penicillamine, corticosteroids and cytostatic drugs. One way of deciding which type of drugs should be given the highest priority in research is to consider the results from controlled clinical trials and select the drugs which have demonstrated ability to cause remission in disease activity and possibly improve the prognosis. This method narrows the field to the stronger acting antirheumatic drugs. Among these I shall discuss three representatives: D-penicillamine, corticosteroids and cytostatic drugs.

Controlled clinical trials have demonstrated that these drugs are able to control disease activity in some of the inflammatory rheumatic diseases. Furthermore we do have some information on the mechanism of action as far as the connective tissue effects are concerned. Finally, their mechanism of action suggest some future lines of connective tissue research in this field.

The process of inflammation includes a large and complicated number of cellular and extracellular phenomena (Willoughby and al. 1977). Probably the anti-inflammatory drugs have different and several sites of action.

The method of evaluation of the mechanism of action of the anti-inflammatory drugs include:
1. Human tissue with rheumatic inflammation, e.g. synovial tissue from rheumatoid joints.
2. Experimental models of rheumatoid inflammation
    A. In vivo models:
        -experimental arthritis
        -experimental granuloma
        -experimental vasculitis
    B. In vitro models:
        -tissue culture

In the following I shall point out some of the connective tissue effects of penicillamine, corticosteroids and cytostatic drugs. The emphasis will be on their effect on the proteoglycans and collagen. Alterations in these components will often reflect the net results of drug effects on the preceding stages of inflammation.

Furthermore, effects on proteoglycans and collagen of uninflammed connective tissue may be of importance to the side effects of the drugs.

D-penicillamine is now widely used in the treatment of

rheumatoid arthritis. It may cause remission in the disease
and perhaps also inhibit cartilage and bone destruction in the
joint. It is characteristic that the effect on the clinical
symptoms of inflammation occurs slowly in the course of 2-4
months or more. Which of penicillamines many biological effects are of importance to its action in rheumatoid arthritis, is unknown (Munthe 1976). The most prominent direct effect on the connective tissue is on collagen. Penicillamine
inhibits the formation of covalent intra- and intermolecular
cross links, and it cleaves also already established cross
links of the aldemine type (Nimni & Bavella 1965, Deshmukh
& Nimni 1969). Furthermore, penicillamine may inhibit the
biosynthesis of collagen (Uitto 1969, Uitto et al. 197o).
These effects have been demonstrated in experimental animal
studies in collagen of granulation tissue, skin, aorta and
bone (Junker et al. 198o, Junker et al. 1981). The effects
are dose-dependant. There is a clear difference in the sensitivity of the collagen of different tissues to the action
of penicillamine, skin collagen being more sensitive than
collagen of granulation tissue. The amount of granulation
tissue seems not to be influenced by penicillamine.

Penicillamine-induced collagen alterations similar to
those in experimental studies have been demonstrated in skin
of patients with rheumatoid arthritis and systemic sclerosis
(Uitto et al. 197o, Hansen TM et al. 1976).

Which are the consequences of the collagen effects of
penicillamine to an anti-inflammatory action? The predomina-
ting effect on collagen in comparison to effects on other
connective tissue components in inflammation suggests that
the early effect of penicillamine on the clinical symptoms
in rheumatoid arthritis must be explained by effects of penicillamine other than those on collagen. However, inhibition of the formation of collagen cross links implies formation of more easily degradable collagen and thereby possibly
an inhibition of fibrosis. In addition cleaving of already
existing labile intermolecular cross links may cause reduction of already established fibrosis. If this assumption is
correct, penicillamine in comparison to other antirheumatic
drugs may be valuable, also in the control of later stages
of inflammation, including fibrosis.

Inhibition or regression of fibrosis may explain the beneficial effect of penicillamine, reported in uncontrolled
studies in systemic sclerosis (Asboe-Hansen 1975). Apart from

the beneficial effects the effect of penicillamine on collagen has important implications as to possible side effects
from long term treatment with penicillamine.

Experimental studies indicate that collagen of non-inflammed connective tissue is more sensitive to the action
of penicillamine than collagen of inflammation. The presence
of cross link deficient collagen in skin, bone and aorta may
imply alterations in the mechanical strength of the tissue.
This have been demonstrated in the skin and aorta of rats
(Oxlund H et al. 1980). Alterations in the mechanical properties of aorta may increase the sensitivity of the artery
to injury, caused by an increased hemodynamic strain similar
to the alterations, observed in some of the hereditary connective tissue diseases, e.g. Marfan's syndrome.

In summary the effects of D-penicillamine on collagen in
granulation tissue may be valuable in controlling the fibrosis in inflammatory rheumatic diseases provided that it is
possible to increase the selectivity i.e. the action on rheumatoid inflammation and decrease the risk of side effects
due to collagen alterations in non-inflammed connective tissue. Possibly, this may be accomplished by combined treatment with other types of antirheumatic drugs.

Glucocorticoids are at present our most powerful and
fastest acting anti-inflammatory drugs. In spite of this the
glucocorticoids have been a disappointment in the treatment
of several of the inflammatory rheumatic diseases. Even if
the glucocorticoids may cause remission in the acute inflammation of rheumatoid arthritis, they are without influence
on bone and cartilage destruction as well as on the ultimate
prognosis. Further, the severe side effects from long term
treatment add another serious chronic disease to the patients
rheumatic disease.

However, at present the glucocorticoids are the most valuable drugs in controlling vasculitis in the rheumatic diseases. Typical examples are giant cell arteritis, in which
corticosteroids may decrease the frequency of complications
such as blindness from about 50% to about 0.

The explanation of the beneficial effects of glucocorticoids in vasculitis is probably that inflammation of the vascular wall frequently is followed by secondary thrombosis
which may lead to irreversible ischemic tissue damage. This

may be prevented by control of vascular inflammation.

One of the main mechanisms of the anti-inflammatory action of the glucocorticoids seems to be an inhibition of the increased vascular permeability of the early stages of inflammation. Thereby the emigration of granulocytes and formation of the early inflammatory exudates is inhibited. The inhibitory action on the increased vascular permeability has been demonstrated in patients with inflammatory rheumatic diseases as well as in experimental studies (Manthorpe et al. 1979 & 1980). Experimental studies have demonstrated that glucocorticoids also inhibit the later stages of inflammation in the vascular wall. The biosynthesis of collagen is inhibited and the degradation is increased, similarly there is an inhibition of the biosynthesis of proteoglycans, RNA and DNA which is stimulated during inflammation and repair in the vascular wall (Manthorpe et al. 1977). Intimal thickening, which is a normal vascular response to injury, is also inhibited. Inhibitory effects similar to those on vascular inflammation have been demonstrated on other types of inflammatory reaction and thus represent a general inhibitory action on non-specific inflammation.

However, the glucocorticoids do have exactly the same type of effects on the proteoglycans and collagen of non-inflammed connective tissue e.g. skin. The effect on non-inflammed connective tissue may explain some of the severe side effects following long term treatment with corticosteroids, such as osteoporosis of the spine, aseptic bone necrosis and vascular purpura. The fact that connective tissue of inflammation is more sensitive to the action of glucocorticoids than non-inflammed connective tissue implies a more favorable effect/side effect ratio as far as the effects on the connective tissue are concerned. This is in contrast to the effect of D-penicillamine on connective tissue.

In conclusion the glucocorticoids are powerful anti-inflammatory drugs, their main advantage being the strong and fast action on inflammation, especially inflammation of the vascular wall. The limitations are the side effects which in part may be explained by the same actions on the connective tissue component involved in the beneficial effects.

Cytostatic drugs have been used in inflammatory rheumatic diseases in severe and otherwise treatment resistant stages. Controlled trials have demonstrated that cytostatic

drugs may cause remission in rheumatoid arthritis. An important advantage seems to be the ability to inhibit cartilage
and bone destruction (Currey et al. 1974). In severe systemic
vasculitis cytostatic drugs in combination with corticosteroids appear to be able to improve survival (Fauci et al.
1979). The cytostatic drugs are used as part of socalled im-
munosuppressive therapy. However, it has not been possible
to demonstrate any parallelism between the inhibitory effects
on the immune system and the effect on the clinical symptoms.
It is therefore likely that an important part of the clinical efficacy of cytostatic drugs is explained by their effects on non-specific mesenchymal reactions.

The effects of cytostatic drugs on non-specific inflammation has been studied in experimental granuloma (Hansen
1979). Cyclophosphamide inhibit the formation of granulation
tissue. This applies to the total amount of granulation tissue as well as to the microscopic constituents of cells and
intercellular substance. Biochemical analysis reveals an inhibition of collagen biosynthesis and collagen degradation.
Similarly, the formation of proteoglycans, RNA and DNA is
inhibited. The alterations in the connective tissue are dose dependant.

In comparison to the effects of the granulation tissue
the influence on a non-inflammed connective tissue is only
small, i.e. the cytostatic drugs have a favorable effect/
side effect ratio as far as the connective tissue is concerned. Their major limitation is the general cytotoxic effect, especially the toxic effect on the bone marrow, which
may imply life threatening side effects.

In conclusion, cytostatic drugs have an inhibitory action on early as well as on late stages of non specific inflammation and repair. Combined treatment with glucocorticoids and cytostatic drugs seems at present to represent our
most powerful anti-inflammatory therapy. The effect/side effect ratio as far as the connective tissue is concerned is
favorable. The risk of serious side effects due to general
cytotoxicity is a major limitation.

FUTURE TRENDS AND PERSPECTIVES

The present knowledge on the etiology and pathogenesis of
the inflammatory rheumatic diseases suggest that non speci-

fic anti-inflammatory therapy will be a necesary part of the
pharmacological control of the diseases. Even at a time,
when the primary etiological factor is identified. A major
problem is to increase the selectivity in order to decrease
the side effects and to increase the efficacy.

A possible strategy may be combination therapy, including
drugs with different points of attack. At present, a combination of anti-inflammatory therapy and immunotherapy, immu-
nosuppression and/or immunostimulation seems to be logical
in several of the inflammatory connective tissue diseases.
Perhaps antimicrobial therapy may also prove rational.

The basis for improvement of the non specific anti-inflammatory treatment is an increased knowledge of the mechanism
of action of the drugs, which in controlled clinical trials
have proved most effective. The differences in the metabolism
of connective tissue of inflammation and non inflammed connective tissue make a favourable effect/side effect ratio
possible as far as the effects on the connective tissue is
concerned. Finally, combination of drugs which act on different points in the process of inflammation and repair may
increase the efficacy and decrease the risk of side effects.

SUMMARY

The primary cause of the most common inflammatory rheumatic
diseases in unknown. Microbial infection combined with an
increased susceptibility due to genetically determined alterations in the immune system is probably of importance. Non-
specific processes of inflammation and repair are the imme-
diate causes of the clinical symptoms, and anti-inflammatory
therapy is at present the corner stone in the control of these diseases. The highest priority in research should be giv-
en to drugs, which in controlled clinical trials have demonstrated ability to cause remission of disease activity. Important examples are D-penicillamine, glucocorticoids and
the cytostatic drugs. The effects of these drugs on the metabolism of proteoglycans and collagen in granulation tissue
and normal connective tissue may explain some of the beneficial effects, but also some of the side effects. Rational
pharmacotherapy in the inflammatory rheumatic diseases may
be a combination of anti-inflammatory drugs with immunotherapy and possibly antimicrobial therapy.

REFERENCES

Asboe-Hansen G (1975). Treatment of generalized scleroderma with inhibitors of connective tissue formation. Acta Dermatovener 55:461.

Currey HLF, Harris J, Mason RM, Woodland J, Beveridge T, Roberts CF, Vera DW, Dixon AStJ, Davis J, Oven Smith B (1974). Comparison of azathioprine, cyclophosphamide and gold in treatment of rheumatoid arthritis. Br Med J 3: 763.

Deshmukh K, Nimni ME (1969). A defect in the intramolecular and intermolecular crosslinking of collagen caused by penicillamine. J Biol Chem 244:1787.

Fauci A, Katz P, Haynes BF, Wolff SM (1979). Cyclophosphamide therapy of severe systemic necrotizing vasculitis. N Engl J Med 3ol:235.

Hansen TM (1979). Cyclophosphamide and collagen. Dan Med Bull 26:45.

Hansen TM, Manthorpe R, Kofod B, Andreassen T, Oxlund H, Lorenzen I (1976). Penicillamine in rheumatoid arthritis. J Rheumatol 3:376.

Junker P, Helin G, Lorenzen I (198o). Effect of D-penicillamine and injury on collagen, glycosaminoglycans, DNA and RNA of granulation tissue and connective tissue of skin, bone and aorta in rats. In preparation.

Junker P, Helin G, Lorenzen I (198o). Effect of different doses of D-penicillamine and combined administration of D-penicillamine and methylprednisolone on collagen, glycosaminoglycans, DNA and RNA of granulation tissue, skin, bone and aorta in rats. In preparation.

Manthorpe R, Garbarsch C, Kofod B, Lorenzen I (1977). Glucocorticoid effects on vascular connective tissue during repair. Acta Endocrinol 86:437.

Manthorpe R, Hansen TM, Junker P, Lorenzen I, Utne HE (1979). Prednisone effect on microvascular permeability in patients with inflammatory rheumatic diseases. Scand J Rheumatol 8:139.

Manthorpe R, Garbarsch C, Lorenzen I (1980). Longterm effect of glucocorticoid on connective tissue of aorta and skin. Acta Endokrinol. In press.

Munthe E (ed. 1976). Penicillamine. Research in rheumatoid disease. Oslo:MSD.

Nimni ME, Bavetta LA (1965). Collagen defect induced by penicillamine. Science 150:905.

Oxlund H, Andreassen TT, Junker P, Lorenzen I (1980). Effect of D-penicillamine and methylprednisolone on the mechanical properties of aorta, skin and tendon in rats. In preparation.

Uitto J (1969). Effect of D-penicillamine on collagen biosynthesis in organ culture. Biochem Biophys Acta 194:498.

Uitto J, Helin P, Rasmussen O, Lorenzen I (1970). Skin collagen in patients with scleroderma. Ann Clin Res 2:228.

Willoughby DA, Giroud JP, Velo GP (eds. 1977). Perspectives in inflammation. Future trends and developments. Lancaster, England: MTP Press Ltd.

Connective Tissue Research:
Chemistry, Biology, and Physiology, Pages 219-223
© 1981 Alan R. Liss, Inc., 150 Fifth Avenue, New York, N.Y. 10011

PHARMACOLOGY OF COLLAGEN

K. Trnavský

Research Institute of Rheumatic Diseases,
Piešťany, Czechoslovakia.

The concept of "collagen diseases" (though misleading)
stimulated vast research of collagen chemistry and physiology. It seems that progressive systemic sclerosis (PSS) is
the only clinical condition among classical diffuse connective tissue diseases which involves detectable disturbance
of collagen metabolism resulting in an increased collagen
deposition (Jayson and Weiss, 1979).

Tissue changes in rheumatoid arthritis could be defined
in terms of overproduction and increased degradation of
collagen. Thus "pharmacology of collagen" has its place
in the field of research devoted to rheumatoid arthritis.
We all know that these tissue changes resulting in the loss
of function are the curse of rheumatoid arthritis. If any
single "new" approach in needed to this problem by those
who search for new basic drugs it can be summarized as looking
at the molecular mechanism of ongoing tissue injury - such
as chondrolysis and pannus formation - and evolving new
methods to find drugs able to preserve the tissues from
further destruction. The attempts to regulate the collagen
production or degradation should be part of this approach
(Trnavská and Trnavský, 1974, Billingham, Lowe, Perry, Turner
and Twose, 1979).

It must be said that all efforts to block the abnormal
synthesis of connective tissue macromolecules including
collagen have been so far unsuccesful. Several methods of
interfering with collagen synthesis in vitro habe been found.
These include methods influencing collagen synthesis through
inhibiting the hydroxylation of collagen, its secretion from

the synthetizing cell, extracellular polymerization etc.
The application of these methods in vivo did not work or was
accompanied by serious problems of side-effects. Some posi-
tive and promising results in controlling abnormal collagen
deposition were gained with penicillamine in PSS (Harris and
Sjoerdsma, 1966, Herbert, Lindberg, Jayson and Bailey, 1974),
liver cirrhosis (Sternlieb, 1975), and rheumatoid arthritis
(Munthe, 1976) (where of course other mechanisms are operating). Another approach is represented by the use of
colchicine which through disrupting microtubules interferes
with collagen synthesis in vitro (Dehm and Prockop, 1972)
and increases secretion of collagenase by cultures of
rheumatoid synovium (Harris and Krane, 1971). One group of
workers has shown colchicine to be effective in the treatment of PSS (Alarcón-Segovia, Ibánez, Kershenobich and Rojkind, 1974) and liver cirrhosis (Rojkind, Uribe and
Kershenobich, 1973). This benefit has not been confirmed by
another study (Gottaduria, Diamond and Kaplan, 1977). In
spite of this authors of colchicine therapy claim its position in the management of PSS (Alarcón-Segovia, 1979) and
others state that its use is based on sound pharmacological
grounds and deserves further full investigation (Rodnan,
1979). Less toxic derivates of colchicine - especially
desacetylcolchiceine - inhibit also collagen biosynthesis
and their clinical application in therapy of fibrosis could
be of practical value (Trnavská, Mikulíková and Trnavský,
1977). Alternative approach to the management of overproduction of collagen is the use of proline analogues which even
in experimental conditions is still controversial (Rojkind,
1973, Dancewicz and Altman, 1974, Chvapil, Madden, Carlson
et al. 1974). Still another agent suggested for basic
therapy of rheumatoid arthritis is levamisole which is
able to inhibit collagen synthesis in vitro (Trnavská, Mikulíková, Trnavský and Rovenský, 1978) and some agents ele-
vating the intracellular level of cAMP are reducing the
amount of newly formed collagen (e.g. theophylline) (Mikulíková, Trnavský and Trnavská, 1980). Steroidal and non-
steroidal antirheumatic drugs may influence the metabolism
of collagen in experimental animal or in vitro and their
actual dosage determine whether stimulation or inhibition
of metabolism is observed (Trnavský, 1974). Any of these
animal experiments can be transposed to clinical practice
only with reservation. Inhibitory effect of many these
drugs is non-specific because they affect not only various
metabolic aspects of collagen but also other steps in the
inflammatory reaction and synthesis of other macromolecules

this could have sometimes deleterious impact e.g. on repara-
tive processes in cartilage).

Increased collagen production in the subsynovial tissue
and joint capsule, invasion of cartilage and subchondral
bone by proliferative mesencymal cells is accompanied by
enzymatic destruction of cartilage by hydrolytic enzymes.
These are products of invasive tissues as well as of leucocytes breaking down in synovial fluid. Collagenolytic
enzymes are part of this enzymatic system operating in active rheumatoid joint. Their number is increasing - apart
from neutral collagenase produced by rheumatoid synovium or
from granulocytes there is evidence of collagenolytic acitity
of cathepsin B1 and neutrophil elastase (Starkey, Barrett
and Burleigh, 1977). Several studies were performed on the
possibility to regulate activity of collagenolytic enzymes
by pharmacological intervention. Some antirheumatic drugs
when tested for their possible inhibition of human leucocyte
collagenase were found to be potent inhibitors. Similarly
some non-steroidal antirheumatic drugs inhibited the collagenolytic activity of cathepsin B1 (Stančíková, Trnavský
and Keilová, 1977). These results speak of course about
"attacking" the final step - already active enzyme. There
are other steps suitable for intervention - the intracellular synthesis of collagenolytic enzymes, their release
and activation of proenzyme. There is recent evidence that
the products of lymphocyte activation could stimulate the
production of neutral collagenase (Dayer et al., 1977).
This could be potential target for cytostatic drugs. Other
possibility is offered by the fact that e.g. leucocytar
collagenase is synthetized as inactive procollagenase. Activating mechanism could be another step accessible to
regulating influences. Pharmacotherapy-sensitive enzymes
(e.g. cathepsin G) have been found to be activators of
latent leucocytar collagenase (Stančíková and Trnavský,1979).

May be that some of these systems should be included
in the preclinical testing and contribute to the search for
a more antietiological agent in the drug therapy of
rheumatoid arthritis.

REFERENCES

Alarcón-Segovia D, Ibánez G, Kershenobich D, Rojkind M (1974).
Treatment of scleroderma. Lancet 1:1054.
Alarcón-Segovia D (1979). Colchicine. Clinics in Rheum.
Dis 5/1:294.
Billingham MEJ, Lowe JS, Perry MA, Turner EH, Twose TM (1979).
Chronic arthritis in rats. The effects of ICI 55, 897.
Abstract of the IXth European Congress of Rheumatology,
Wiesbaden.
Chvapil M, Madden JW, Carlson EC et al. (1974). Effect of
cis-hydroxyproline on collagen and other proteins in skin
wounds, granuloma tissue and liver of mice and rats. Exp
Mol Pathol 20:363.
Dancewicz AM, Altman KI (1974). The effect of azetidine-2-
carboxylic acid on the bioxynthesis of collagen in rat
granuloma. Acta Biochim Polonica 21:429.
Dayer JM et al. (1977). Collagenase production by rheumatoid
synovial cells: Stimulation by human lymphocyte factor.
Science 195:181.
Dehm P, Prockop JD (1972). Time lang in the secretion of
collagen by matrix-free tendon cells and inhibition of
the secretory process by colchicine and vinblastine.
Biochim Biophys Acta 264:375.
Gottaduria M, Diamond H, Kaplan D (1977). Colchicine in the
treatment of scleroderma. J Rheumatol 4:272.
Harris ED, Sjoerdsma A (1966). Effect of penicillamine on
human collagen and its possible application to treatment
of scleroderma. Lancet 2:996.
Harris ED, Krane SM (1971). Effects of colchicine on collagenase in cultures of rheumatoid synovium. Arthr Rheum
14:669.
Herbert C, Lindberg KA, Jayson MIV, Bailey AJ (1974).
Scleroderma: Biosynthesis and maturation of skin collagen
and the effects of D-penicillamine. Lancet 1:187.
Jayson MIV, Weiss JB (1979). Progressive systemic sclerosis:
Metabolism of connective tissue. Clinics in Rheum Dis
5/1:185.
Mikulíková D, Trnavský K, Trnavská Z (1980). Influence of
aminophylline on biosynthesis of collagen and non-collagen
proteins, in vitro. Int J Tiss Reac 2:15.
Munthe E (ed) (1976). Penicillamine research in rheumatoid
arthritis. Proceedings of a Symposium held at Spatind,
Norway.
Rodnan GP (1979). Foreword. Clinics in Rheum Dis 5/1:1.

Rojkind M (1973). Inhibition of liver fibrosis by 1-azetidine-2-carboxylic acid in rats treated with carbon tetrachloride. J Clin Invest 52:2451.

Rojkind M, Uribe M, Kershenobich D (1973). Colchicine and treatment of liver fibrosis. Lancet 1:38.

Stančíková M, Trnavský K (1979). Activation of latent collagenase from polymorphonuclear leucocytes by cathepsin G. Collection 44:3177.

Stančíková M, Trnavský, Keilová H (1977). The effect of antirheumatic drugs on collagenolytic activity of cathepsin B1. Biochem Pharmacol 26:2121.

Starkey PM, Barrett AJ, Burleigh MC (1977). The degradation of articular collagen by neutrophil proteinases. Biochim Biophys Acta 483:386.

Sternlieb I (1975). Penicillamine and hepatic fibrosis. In Popper H, Becker K (eds): Collagen metabolism in the liver. New York: Stratton Intercontinental Medical Book Corp.

Trnavská Z, Mikulíková D, Trnavský K, Rovenský J (1978). Wirkung von Levamisol auf die Kollagensynthese in vitro. Z Rheumatol 37/38:221.

Trnavská Z, Mikulíková D, Trnavský K (1977). The effect of colchicine and its derivatives on the collagen biosynthesis in vitro. Agents and Actions 7:563.

Trnavská Z, Trnavský K (1974). Influence of nonsteroidal antirheumatic drugs on collagen metabolism in rats with adjuvant-induced arthritis. Pharmacology 12:110.

Trnavský K (1974). Some effects of antiinflammatory drugs on connective tissue metabolism. In Scherrer R, Whitehouse MW (eds). Antiinflammatory agents, vol. II. New York: Academic Press.

Connective Tissue Research:
Chemistry, Biology, and Physiology, Pages 225–231
© **1981 Alan R. Liss, Inc., 150 Fifth Avenue, New York, N.Y. 10011**

REGULATION OF CONNECTIVE TISSUE PROTEASES

F.S. Steven

Department of Medical Biochemistry,
Stopford Building, University of Manchester,
Manchester M13 9PT
England

1. INTRODUCTION

The term connective tissue protease could be defined as
any protease which may be shown to degrade one or more of
the protein components of connective tissue such as the core
protein of proteoglycans, collagen fibrils or elastin fibres.
The term could equally well be used to define protease which
may be present in connective tissues, either intra- or extracellularly. It therefore seems best to consider regulation
of protease activity in rather general terms since the par-
ticipants in this workshop have interpreted this title rather
liberally. Much of the work to be discussed concerns the
control of protease activity through inhibitors and in some
cases the regain of enzymic actvity by disulphide exchange.
In this outline of regulatory mechanisms, I have tried to
place a reference to each of the submitted abstracts in the
most appropriate section. It is hoped that other work will
be presented by those who have not submitted abstracts.

2. REGULATION BY ZYMOGEN ACTIVATION

Control of proteolysis can be exerted by the activation
of a proenzyme or zymogen; for example the activation of
collagenase from procollagenase reported by Harper, Block
and Gross (1971) and the well-known plasminogen activation
system converting plasminogen to plasmin. Both these
processes require the presence of a suitable activating
protease to initiate activation of the proenzymes. The
whole process may be blocked by the presence of inhibitor(s)

for either the activating enzyme or for the newly-formed
product of activation, ie. collagenase or plasmin in the
above example. In this regard it is of interest that plasmin,
a protease very similar to trypsin, is not inhibited by the
seven trypsin inhibitors present in whole blood (Heimburger,
1974), otherwise the physiological resorption of a fibrin
clot would not be possible. It also follows that the
plasminogen activator system is not inhibited by these
protease inhibitors present in whole blood, such as α_2-macro-
globulin which has a very wide specificity for inhibition of
proteases (Barratt and Starkey, 1973).

3. REGULATION BY RELEASE OF LYSOSOMAL ENZYMES

The release of lysosomal enzymes (eg. Cathepsin D,
Dingle, Barratt and Poole, 1972) has been shown to promote
the destruction of cartilage, although the physiological
regulation of the export of lysosomal enzymes appears complex.
Dr. Fabry will present evidence on the effect of experimental
haemarthrosis on the degradation of cartilage proteoglycans
attributed to the release of cathepsin D. The substrate
specificities of three arginine aminopeptidases which are
released from leucocytes during phagocytosis will be described by Dr. Söderling. The activity of lysosomal enzymes
in synoviocytes and chondrocytes during inflammation will
be described by Dr. Henderson whilst the effect of exercise
on the activity of cartilage lysosomal enzymes will be described by Drs. Kiiskinen, Pekki and Tauriainen.

When considering lysosomal enzymes in the extracellular
environment it is important to remember that the control of
their activity is exercised at two levels (a) the actual
release of these enzymes by the cell and (b) the pH of the
extracellular fluid which is normally much higher than the
pH optimum of most lysosomal proteases.

4. REGULATION BY ACTIVE SITE DIRECTED PROTEASE INHIBITORS

Most inhibitors of proteases require to possess a compli-
mentary structure on part of the inhibitor molecule which
fits the active centre of the protease. Enzyme and inhibitor
molecules interact to form an enzyme-inhibitor complex, eg.
trypsin and soybean trypsin inhibitor are typical of this
class of interactants. This selectivity of interaction may

be conveniently applied for the isolation of both pure enzymes and pure inhibitors employing affinity chromatography techniques. The inhibition of granulocyte proteases by inhibitors isolated from colostrum and seminal fluid will be described by Drs Stančiková, Čechová and Trnavský. Drs. Hurych, Miřejovská and Kobrle will describe the decrease in activity of PZ-peptidase in the lungs of animals with experimental silicotic fibrosis.

5. REGULATION BY α_2-MACROGLOBULIN

Barratt and Starkey (1973) demonstrated the ability of α_2-macroglobulin to complex with a large number of proteases in a stoichiometric manner following the cleavage of a single peptide bond within the α_2-macroglobulin. It is thought that the proteolytic enzymes are trapped within the α_2-macroglobulin and that the enzyme-α_2M-complex is destined for phagocytic digestion. Mammalian collagenase is a remarkably specific enzyme in the fact that it cleaves only three peptide bonds in the intact tropocollagen monomer, yet the enzyme is also inhibited by α_2-macroglobulin (Werb, Burleigh, Barratt and Starkey, 1974). One of the other unusual properties of α_2-macroglobulin complexes with proteases is that the enzyme appears to be active within the complex, provided that the substrate can gain access to the enzyme. Small substrates are still cleaved at much the same rate as by the unbound enzyme, we should therefore consider circulating α_2-M-enzyme-complexes as functional enzymes.

6. REGULATION BY KUNITZ TYPE OF INHIBITORS

Low molecular weight inhibitors of a wide variety of proteases such as the Kunitz inhibitor or trasylol are commonly found in the extracellular matrix. These inhibitors have molecular weights of approximately 6000 daltons. Cartilage has been shown to contain an inhibitor of trypsin by Kuettner, Hiti, Eisenstein and Harper (1976) having molecular weight of 12000 daltons. Rifkin and Crowe (1977) isolated a similar inhibitor from cartilage and aorta with a molecular weight of 6000 daltons, this molecule was shown to be identical with trasylol and it was observed to chromatograph as a dimer with molecular weight of 12000-13000 daltons. Three inhibitors of molecular weight approximately 13000 daltons will be described by Drs. Brzin, Giraldi, Kopitar and Turk during this workshop. These inhibitors were shown to produce significant reduction in spontaneous lung metastases in mice bearing Lewis lung carcinoma.

Dr. Anderson will describe studies on the inhibitors of proteolytic enzymes present in aorta and cartilage extracts. He will draw attention to the ability of proteoglycans to bind an undegraded isotopically labelled protein substrate in the presence of trichloroacetic acid, thus leading to a methodological hazard in the assay of proteases by the technique described by Peterkofsky and Diegelmann (1971). The theory and practical details of incremental analysis (Steven, Podrazký and Foster, 1978) will be developed by Dr. Podrazký.

7. REGULATION BY DISULPHIDE EXCHANGE

The active centre of trypsin (and also chymotrypsin and elastase) is maintained in the correct conformation for the expression of enzymic activity by a disulphide bond located on either side of the sequence which comprises a major portion of the active centre (Nights and Light, 1976). An inhibitor of trypsin was obtained from Ehrlich ascites tumour cells (Steven and Podrazký, 1978) and it was demonstrated that the inhibitor possessed a reactive thiol which interacted with the significant disulphide bond of trypsin. The reaction could be mimicked with synthetic thiols and reversed by cystine, TPCK-chymotrypsin and chymotrypsinogen (Steven and Podrazký, 1979). Biphasic re-activation and inhibition was demonstrated with mersalyl (Steven, Podrazký and Itzhaki, 1978) and metal ions (Steven, Podrazký, Al-Habib and Griffin, 1979). A model system involving sequential treatment of trypsin and chymotrypsin with thiols followed by incremental additions of $NaIO_4$ also demonstrated biphasic re-activation and inhibition of these enzymes (Steven and Al-Habib, 1979). From these studies it was clear that a reversible thiol disulphide interaction took place as follows:

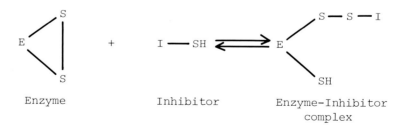

| Enzyme | Inhibitor | Enzyme-Inhibitor complex |

In this workshop the details of organomercurial re-activation of latent enzymes will be developed in depth (Steven and Griffin, 1980). Mersalyl has been extensively used to activate latent collagenase by Sellers, Cartwright, Murphy and Reynolds (1977) and by Sellers and Reynolds (1977). It was therefore of particular interest that Macartney and Tschesche (1980) demonstrated that latency was due to the presence of a thiol-containing inhibitor linked by an inter-molecular disulphide bond to collagenase. This study will be presented in the workshop.

8. REGULATION OF A SPECIFIC ENZYME BY A SPECIFIC INHIBITOR

The most appropriate example of this type of interaction is the specific inhibitor for mammalian collagenase described by Woolley, Glanville, Robertson and Evanson (1978).

9. PROPERTIES OF CELL SURFACE NEUTRAL PROTEASES

Ehrlich ascites tumour cells possess a trypsin-like enzyme on their surface which is inhibited by active site titrants for trypsin and active site directed agents such as TLCK, p-aminobenzamidine etc., but the surface enzyme is not inhibited by trasylol or protein inhibitors of trypsin in free solution. The enzyme is involved in the activation of both tumour-exported procollagenase and plasma-derived plasminogen, and could therefore be important in controlling the invasive properties of tumour cells. Model experiments with trypsin-Sepharose indicate that trypsin-like enzymes attached to surfaces are protected from the approach of high molecular weight inhibitors of trypsin. It can be concluded that cell-surface-bound proteases must be considered in a different light to our understanding of control mechanisms which have been elucidated for the same enzymes in free solution.

Barratt AJ, Starkey PM (1973). Interaction of α_2-macro-globulin with proteinases. Biochem J 133:709.
Dingle JT, Barratt AJ, Poole AR (1972). Inhibition by pepstatin of human cartilage degradation. Biochem J 127:443.
Harper E, Block KJ, Gross J (1971). The zymogen of tadpole collagenase. Biochemistry 10:3033.

Heimburger N (1974). Biochemistry of proteinase inhibitors from human plasma: a review of recent development. In Fritz H, Tschesche H, Greene LJ, Truscheit E (eds): "Proteinase Inhibitors", Bayer-Symposium V New York: Springer-Verlag, p 14.

Kuettner KE, Hiti J, Eisenstein R, Harper E (1976). Collagenase inhibition by cationic proteins derived from cartilage and aorta. Biochem Biophys Res Comm 72:40.

Macartney HW, Tschesche H (1980). Latent collagenase from human polymorphonuclear leucocytes and activation to collagenase by removal of an inhibitor. Febs letters (in press).

Nights RJ, Light A (1976). Disulphide bond modified trypsinogen. J Biol Chem 251:222.

Peterkofsky B, Diegelmann (1971). Use of a mixture of proteinase-free collagenases for the specific assay of radioactive collagen in the presence of other proteins. Biochemistry 10:988.

Rifkin DB, Crowe RM (1977). Isolation of a protease from tissues resistant to tumour invasion. Hoppe Seyler's Z Physiol Chem 358:1525.

Sellers A, Cartwright E, Murphy G, Reynolds JJ (1977). Evidence that latent collagenases are enzyme inhibitor complexes. Biochem J 163:303.

Sellers A, Reynolds JJ (1977). Identification and partial characterisation of an inhibitor of collagenase from rabbit bones. Biochem J 167:353.

Steven FS, Al-Habib A (1979). Inhibition of trypsin and chymotrypsin by thiols. Biphasic kinetics of re-activation and inhibition induced by sodium periodate addition. Biochim Biophys Acta 568:408.

Steven FS, Griffin MG (1980). Studies on the molecular mechanism of mersalyl and 4-aminophenylmercuric acetate re-activation of trypsin-thiol complexes. Eur J Biochem (in press).

Steven FS, Podrazký V (1978). Evidence for the inhibition of trypsin by thiols. The mechanism of enzyme-inhibitor complex formation. Eur J Biochem 83:155.

Steven FS, Podrazký V (1979). The reversible thiol-disulphide exchange of trypsin and chymotrypsin with a tumour derived inhibitor. Kinetic data obtained with fluorescein-labelled polymeric collagen fibrils and casein as substrates. Biochim Biophys Acta 568:49.

Steven FS, Podrazký V, Al-Habib A, Griffin MM (1979). Biphasic kinetics of metal ion re-activation of trypsin-thiol complexes. Biochim Biophys Acta 571:369.

Steven FS, Podrazký V, Foster RW (1978). Incremental analysis: the application to quantitation of both enzyme activity and inhibitory activity in complex subcellular fractions. Anal Biochem 90:183.

Steven FS, Podrazký V, Itzhaki S (1978). The interaction of a trypsin-dependent neutral protease and its inhibitor found in tumour cells. Biochim Biophys Acta 524:170.

Werb Z, Burleigh MC, Barratt AJ, Starkey PM (1974). The interaction of α_2-macroglobulin with proteases. Biochem J 139:359.

Woolley DE, Glanville RW, Robertson DR, Evanson JM (1978). Purification, characterisation and inhibition of human skin collagenase. Biochem J 169:265.

Connective Tissue Research:
Chemistry, Biology, and Physiology, Pages 233–246
© **1981 Alan R. Liss, Inc., 150 Fifth Avenue, New York, N.Y. 10011**

CONTROL OF ELASTIC TISSUE DESTRUCTION BY ELASTASE INHIBITORS

HORNEBECK W., BELLON G., BRECHEMIER D., GODEAU G., ROBERT L.

Laboratoire de Biochimie du Tissu Conjonctif (GR CNRS N° 40)
Faculté de Médecine, 8 rue du Général Sarrail
94010 Créteil-Cedex, France

INTRODUCTION

It is generally accepted that the disturbance of the protease-protease inhibitor balance can lead to protease mediated tissue destruction, such mechanisms being involved in the genesis of pathological processes (Dingle, 1978 ; Bieth, 1978 ; Eriksson, 1978).

Elastic tissue degradation was considered to be due only to elastase(s) because of the great resistance of elastin to most proteolytic enzymes at neutral pH. In vitro experiments indicated that hydrolysis of elastin by elastase(s) was influenced, among other factors, by the adsorption of the enzyme on to its substrate and by the accessibility of specific bonds susceptible to cleavage (Hornebeck, 1980).

Elastolysis is also under the control of naturally occuring inhibitors originated from the plasma and/or the tissues (Bieth, 1978). Nevertheless, we want to present, here, evidences in favor of the contention that plasma inhibitors e.g. α_1-proteinase inhibitor (α_1PI) and α_2-macroglobulin (α_2M) may not be always efficient in controlling elastic tissue destruction by elastase(s). We also want to discuss the potential therapeutic value of elastase inhibitors in diseases of elastic tissues.

I - INTERACTIONS BETWEEN ELASTASE(S) AND ENDOGENOUS INHIBI-
TORS

α_1-proteinase inhibitor (also called α_1-antitrypsin)
and α_2-macroglobulin are the two important elastase inhibitors present in human plasma. Neither is specific for inhibiting elastase(s) since α_1PI possesses a broad spectrum of
inhibition on serine proteases (Morse, 1978) and α_2M inhibits all endopeptidases (Starkey and Barrett, 1977).

α_1 Proteinase Inhibitor

α_1PI is present at a relatively high concentration in
human serum ($\sim$ 25 μM) and in contrast with α_2M is an acute
phase protein (Laurell, 1972). Reaction of α_1PI with serine
proteases involves the cleavage of a peptide bond within the
inhibitor molecule (Cohen et al., 1978). In the case of
elastase (from leucocytes) it has been reported that this
reaction resulted in a rapid inactivation of α_1PI by the
enzyme (Baumstark et al., 1977). Elastase(s) and α_1PI react
stoechiometrically and both the esterolytic and elastinolytic activities of the enzyme are abolished in the complex
(Bellon et al., 1979). Kinetic studies have indicated that
the inhibition of elastase by α_1PI may be described by an
irreversible second order process and the transfer of enzyme
from α_1PI complexes to free α_2M was not observed (Bieth,
1978).

Nevertheless, elastolysis was found to occur even after
effective complex formation and the temporary character of
the inhibition of elastase(s) by α_1PI in presence of elastin
has to be envisaged (Martin and Taylor, 1979).

As "avidity" of elastase(s) for elastin may be greater
than for α_1PI, dissociation of the α_1PI-elastase complexes
could be facilitated at the vicinity of elastic fibers.

Deficiency of α_1PI may be genetically determined or it
may be functional as a result of the "consumption" of inhibitor by chemical or enzymatic mechanisms.

To date about 20 phenotypes of human α_1PI have been
identified. Individuals of the PiZZ and PiSZ genotypes (slow
moving electrophoretic forms) have much lower amounts of
α_1PI in their plasma. Consequently they were found highly
susceptible to juvenile chronic lung disease (Eriksson,
1978).

Cystein active site proteinases (papain, Cathepsin B_1) have been found to inactivate α_1PI by proteolytic cleavage of a scissile peptide bond. As a result altered levels of this endopeptidase may well disrupt the balance between elastase(s) and α_1PI. Hydrogen cyanide, present in cigaret smoke activates thiol proteinases and may be one of the prime agents of the induction of elastolysis in lung tissue (Johnson and Travis, 1977).

Recently other investigations have shown that oxidizing agents can block the elastase-inhibitory activity of human α_1PI by oxidizing a critical methionine residue present in the active site of the inhibitor molecule (Johnson and Travis, 1979). The trypsin inhibitory activity of α_1PI was unaffected and such effect can be reproduced by in vivo experiments by intravenous injection of a large dose of chloramine T into monkeys. Cohen found a marked decrease in elastase inhibitory activity which was restored to its original level after 3.7 days (Cohen, 1979).

Determination of the antielastase activity of α_1PI of smokers and non-smokers indicated a nearly two fold reduction in the functional activity of this particular inhibitor in the lungs of cigaret smokers (Crystal, 1980).

In our laboratory, we determined the elastase inhibitory capacity of the sera of smokers and non-smokers. We found that it decreases with the age of the individuals, independently from smoking habits. Nevertheless, this decrease was more pronounced in smokers, the difference between both groups being significant (Robert et al., 1980). As immunologically reactive α_1-antiprotease and α_2M was found nearly invariant with age, the loss of inhibitory capacity we observed may be interpreted as a dysfunctionality of the serum inhibitors with aging. Such decrease was accelerated with smoking habits and may reflect the partial inactivation of α_1PI by cigaret oxidizing agents or other factors. This mechanism may partly be responsible for the slow fragmentation and disappearance of elastic lamellae occuring in most individuals with aging.

α_2-Macroglobulin (α_2M)

Binding of α_2M with proteinases has been thoroughly studied by many investigators (Starkey and Barrett, 1977 ; Harpel, 1976).

It can be stated that catalytically active forms of all endopeptidases react with α_2M and the enzyme may be considered as irreversibly bound. Furthermore, competition experiments with several proteases indicated that saturation of α_2M molecules with one protease prevents the binding of other proteases. α_2M cannot be considered as a typical protease inhibitor since inhibition of enzyme activity only resulted in the steric hindrance of the protease active site in the complex. We have determined that α_2M-porcine pancreatic elastase kept 73.5 % of the activity of free enzyme on Suc-(Ala)$_3$-pna*. The activity of such complexes is much lower on protein substrates but a well defined activity could be demonstrated towards soluble forms of elastin composed of peptides of high molecular weights (Robert et al., 1980). Such complexes retained a small but detectable activity towards SDS treated insoluble elastin also.

Contrarily to α_1PI-elastase complexes, α_2M-elastase complexes are quickly eliminated from the circulation with a half-time of less than 10 minutes, being phagocytosed by the cells of the reticuloendothelial system (Ohlsson and Laurell, 1976).

In normal circumstances, the residual elastinolytic activity of α_2M-elastase(s) complexes cannot be expressed since escape of such complexes from the circulation is highly improbable due to their rapid clearance and high molecular weight. Nevertheless in conditions where tissue permeability increases, such as during hypertension, hypercholesterolemia, inflammatory processes, α_2M-elastase(s) may well escape from the circulation and penetrate connective tissues (vessel walls, etc) and express their proteolytic action.

We demonstrated an elastinolytic activity in human sera (Bellon et al., 1978) and the presence of circulating elastase(s) was reported by other authors (Geokas et al., 1977). The activity hydrolysing Suc-(Ala)$_3$-pna was found equivalent to 40 ng of porcine pancreatic elastase per ml of serum ; more than 80 per cent of this activity was precipitable by anti-α_2-macroglobulin antibodies. As it was found that in man approximately 10 per cent of the circulating α_2M is catabolized each day, the significance of such elastase activity probably bound to α_2M molecules needs to be further investigated.

* Succinoyl trialanyl paranitroanilide

Other Examples of Inhibitory Deficiency Related to Elastin
Catabolism

The two most studied elastases are pancreatic and leukocyte elastases but other elastinolytic enzymes have been
isolated from macrophages and platelets (De Cremoux et al.,
1978 ; Hornebeck et al., 1980). We recently evidenced the
presence of elastase-type proteases in several mesenchymal
cells including aortic smooth muscle cells (from rat and
pig origin) and human fibroblasts (skin, vulva)(Bourdillon
et al., 1980). These isolated enzymes possessed much lower
activity on insoluble elastin than pancreatic or leukocyte
elastases but could nevertheless induce an important degradation of elastic fibers when injected subcutaneously to
young rabbits (Godeau et al., in prep.). In tissue culture
experiments however, we could not detect any elastase activity in serum free culture medium from aortic smooth muscle
cells or human fibroblasts. The whole enzyme activity was
in each case extractible from cells with buffers containing
Triton-X-100. To date, we have no information on the possible in vivo extracellular release of such elastase-type
proteases in catabolic situations. If such enzymes are indeed
excreted from these cells, it is highly probable that the
local concentration of proteases would exceed the concentration of preexisting plasma inhibitors. We recently demonstrated that inhibition of leukocyte elastase by human α_1PI
was about 50 per cent suppressed if the proteinase was first
preincubated with elastin prior to addition of the inhibitor
(Hornebeck and Schnebli, 1980). This finding indicates that
α_1PI but also probably α_2M could not effectively control
elastic tissue destruction as soon as elastase(s) reached
first elastic fibers.

We will now describe two other examples of the ineffi-
ciency of α_1PI and/or α_2M in controlling elastic tissue
degradation. The most obvious one concerns elastolytic proteases classified as metallo-proteinases which are inhibited
by α_2M but whose enzymatic activity is unaffected by α_1PI.
As examples, we will first mention the elastase-like protease
we and other investigators have isolated from macrophages
(Werb and Gordon, 1975 ; De Cremoux et al., 1978). We determined that the activity hydrolyzing elastin of 1 mg of
enzyme in a partially purified form (isolated from monkey
alveolar macrophages) was fully inhibited by 11 ml of human
serum as compared with 1.1 ml of the same serum employing
the same amount of porcine pancreatic elastase. We also
found that significantly higher elastase amounts were secreted by cells when exposed to latex or zymosan as was reported

Table 1

Elastase activity in different cells.

The enzyme was extracted from cells with 0.1M tris-HCl pH 8.0 containing 0.1 % Triton-X-100. The results are expressed as µg porcine pancreatic elastase equivalents on Suc-(Ala)$_3$-pna per 10^{10} cells ; they represented the mean of at least 3 separate determinations.

Cells	Elastase activity
Human polymorphonuclear neutrophils	1440
Monkey alveolar macrophages	116.2
Human blood platelets	7.8
Human skin fibroblasts	65.2
Human vulva fibroblasts	836
Rat aorta smooth muscle cells	5.6
Rat skin fibroblasts	22.4
Human cancer cells (MCF 7)	18.1

for murine macrophages when exposed to cigaret smoke (White et al., 1979). These results tend to support the concept that macrophage elastase may be as important as leukocyte elastase in the destruction of (lung) elastin. It has to be emphasized however, that macrophages may act in a bifunctional manner during elastic tissue destruction: first in a catabolic way by secreting an elastase-like protease,but also in a protective manner as it has been reported that leukocyte elastase binds rapidly to alveolar macrophages in vitro and further incorporated into phagolysosomes. As this binding did not require α_2M, macrophages may well have a clearance role for lysosomal elastase at tissue sites where plasma inhibitors are present only at a low level or in case of a dysfunctionality of α_1PI (Campbell et al., 1979).

Another elastase-type metallo-protease we will also shortly discuss is the enzyme we recently isolated from fibroblasts obtained from human vulva-tissue. This enzyme hydrolysed maximally Suc-(Ala)$_3$-pna and MeO-Suc-(Ala)$_2$-Pro Val-pna around pH 8.0, was inactivated by EDTA. It was found to be fully reactivated by calcium ions (Frances et al., in prep.).

As a second main escape mechanism from the inhibitory control of elastase(s), lipoprotein-bound elastase activities have to be mentioned. We found that an activity hydrolysing rhodamine labeled insoluble elastin and Suc-(Ala)$_3$-pna was associated with VLDL (Very Low Density Lipoproteins d<1.0068), LDL (Low Density Lipoproteins 1.0068<d<1.063) and also HDL (High Density Lipoproteins 1.063<d<1.21) fractions of human serum. HDL fractions contained the higher activity which represented 4 to 23 per cent (depending on the serum) of the total enzymatic activity of human serum. Contrarily to the elastase activity bound to VLDL which was inhibited by active site serine protease inhibitors (Pmsf ; DipF), the partially purified protease from HDL fractions by Lima bean trypsin inhibitor affinity chromatography appeared to be a metallo-proteinase as indicated by its inhibition by metal chelating agents (1,10-phenanthrolin, EDTA). In the complex form with the lipoproteins the elastase(s)-type protease was not affected by plasma inhibitors (α_1PI and α_2M). Furthermore porcine pancreatic elastase added to human serum did not seem to bind to lipoproteins to any detectable extent. As lipoproteins were shown to penetrate easily the arterial wall, the physiological importance of such elastase-lipoprotein complexes in arteriosclerosis should not be underestimated (Robert et al., 1980).

II - EXOGENOUS INHIBITORS AS A POSSIBLE TOOL FOR CONTROLLING
ELASTIC TISSUE DESTRUCTION.

In the case of an altered level or a dysfunctionality
of elastase inhibitors it could be reasonably assumed that
the balance between elastases and antielastases may be
artificially and temporarily restored by adding exogenous
inhibitors to the system as a therapeutic approach.

A suitable inhibitor to a particular proteolytic enzyme
must satisfy a number of conditions which have been reviewed
by Knight (1977) and Lawson (1978).

The essential requirement of lack of antigenicity of
the compound excludes a priori large molecules with the
exception of α_1PI which has been used in some cases for the
in vivo suppression of elastase induced emphysema in animals
(Yoshida and Shiu Yeh Yu, 1979) and is under clinical investigations also (Crystal et al., 1980). However we previously
mentioned that once bound to elastin elastase was partially
refractory to its natural inhibitor. Furthermore its utilisation is limited to the inhibition of serine proteases
(leukocyte, pancreatic elastases) and will be completely
unsatisfactory in the case of an increased level of macrophage elastase or against the Pseudomonas aeruginosa elastase (both are metallo-proteases)(Nishino and Powers, 1980).

Low molecular weight synthetic inhibitors have been
synthesized. Both reversible and irreversible inhibitors
were designed by analogy with their best synthetic substrates taking into account the extended substrate binding sites
for both proteases. The best known are the peptide-chloro-
methylketones (Powers et al., 1977), some of them exhibited
excellent specificites and efficiencies but have the disad-
vantage of presenting toxicity. They were used, however,
quite successfully in emphysema therapy. Stone et al. found
a moderation of (0.1 mg) elastase induced emphysema in
hamsters by a treatment (1 hour later) with 0.5 mg of
Suc-(Ala)$_2$-Pro-Val-chloromethylketone as indicated by a
much lower value of quasi-static lung compliance (Stone et
al., 1979).

Reversible elastase inhibitors have been isolated from
the filtrates of cultures of Streptomyces:Elasnin (from
Streptomyces noboritoensis)(Omura et al., 1979) and Elastatinal (from Streptomyces griseoruber)(Umezawa and Aoyagi,
1977). Elasnin markedly inhibits human granulocyte elastase
but was found far less active towards porcine pancreatic

elastase. The K_i values for elastatinal (peptide aldehyde) have been determined for pancreatic and leukocyte elastases (Feinstein et al., 1976). They were respectively equal to 2.10^{-7}M and 5.10^{-5}M and again this compound has been used to reduce experimentally induced elastase-emphysema (Yoshida and Yu, 1979).

Desmosines (White et al., 1979) and bovine Kunitz pancreatic inhibitor (Trasylol)(Lestienne and Bieth, 1978) have been reported to inhibit elastase(s) in vitro and Nishino and Powers (1980) recently synthesized synthetic peptide derivatives which inhibited Pseudomonas aeruginosa elastase (a metallo-elastase also able, as cathepsin B_1, to inactivate α_1PI).

Finally two protease inhibitors, eglins isolated from the Leech Hirudo medicinalis were found to inhibit elastase(s) with very low dissociation constants (Seemüller et al., 1977). In contrast with α_1PI we recently showed that methoxy-succinyl-$(Ala)_2$-Pro-Val-chloromethylketone and eglin C inactivated human leukocyte elastase nearly completely, regardless of whether or not the enzyme was adsorbed to its substrate elastin prior to the addition of the inhibitors (Hornebeck and Schnebli, submitted). Eglin C may also provide an in vivo protection against preadsorbed elastase as indicated by data shown on Figure 1.

In this experiment, we injected subcutaneously to a 3 weeks old rabbit either leukocyte elastase (100 µg) or the same amount of active enzyme followed by the administration of eglin C at the same site, one hour after the injection of the elastase ; 6 hours later, the states of both local epidermis elastic fibers were compared to those of control animals which received either physiological saline or Pmsf inactivated enzyme. This experiment was repeated twice (with other young rabbits) and the quantitative expression of the results were done by screen enlargement of stained sections (orcein treated) and computer analysis (Godeau et al., in prep.). The mean lenght of epidermal elastic fibers was found equal to 220 + 40 arbitrary units (A.U.), 88 + 42 and 170 + 37 respectively for controls, elastase treated, elastase and eglin C treated animals. The differences were highly significant between elastase treated and control animals but were not significant between control animals and those which received a subcutaneous injection of eglin C after the injection of leukocyte elastase.

As concluding remarks it should be stated that the

Figure 1

In vivo degradation of rabbit skin (3 weeks old) elastic
fibers by human leukocyte elastase. Protection effect of
eglin C. Rabbit skin thin sections were stained by orcein
treatment (Godeau et al., in prep.). Magnification x 1000
EF = elastic fibers.

Skin (epidermis) elastic fibers appearance 6 hours after :
1 - (Control experiment) subcutaneous injection of 100 μg of
    Pmsf inactivated leukocyte elastase.
2 - (Treated animals) subcutaneous injection of 100 μg of
    active leukocyte elastase.
3 - (Treated animals) subcutaneous injection of 100 μg of
    active leukocyte elastase (0.5 ml) followed by injection
    (1 hour after at the same site) of 50 μg (0.5 ml) of
    eglin C.

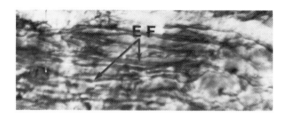

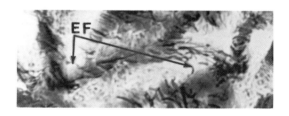

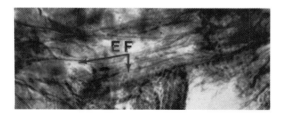

proper use of any inhibitor obviously needs the knowledge of the precise nature of the enzyme (elastase(s))responsible for elastin degradation during the course of a particular pathological event. In lung diseases for instance at least 3 elastase(s) or elastinolytic enzymes (originated from leukocytes, macrophages and/or mesenchymal cells) may well be involved (separately or in a cumulative fashion) in elastin catabolism. In arteriosclerosis the source of aorta elastin degrading enzymes can also be multiple. Ideally a bifunctional elastase inhibitor may be designed ; one part of the molecule presenting an affinity for the elastin substrate and the other part exhibiting a broad specificity for elastin degrading proteases. Such compounds could even be used in a preventive treatment.

So far, elastase(s) were considered to possess only negative metabolic functions. They may however participate in other biological processes as, for instance, in regulating cyclic AMP levels. Porcine pancreatic elastase was found effective in stimulating adenylate cyclase activity (Lacombe et al., 1979). Results obtained in human breast tumors also suggested that elastolytic proteases may be involved in the processing of freshly synthesised elastin or in some other processes correlated to the biosynthesis of elastin (Hornebeck et al., 1978).

We have not mentioned several other ways of controlling elastic fiber destruction by regulating the amount of endogenous tissue inhibitors, the synthesis of elastin or even the "catabolic factors" responsible of elastase secretion by cells.

REFERENCES

Baumstark JS, Ting Lee C, Luby RJ (1977). Rapid inactivation of α_1-protease inhibitor (α_1-antitrypsin) by elastase. Biochim Biophys Acta 482:400.

Bellon G, Hornebeck W, Derouette JC, Robert L (1978). Méthodes simples pour quantifier l'élastase et ses inhibiteurs dans le sérum humain. Pathol Biol 26:515.

Bieth J (1978). Elastases : structure, function and pathological role. In Robert L (ed): "Frontiers of Matrix Biology," Basel: Karger, 6:1.

Bourdillon MC, Brechemier D, Blaes N, Derouette JC, Hornebeck W, Robert L (1980). Elastase-like enzymes in skin fibroblasts and rat aorta smooth muscle cells. Cell Biol Int Rep 4:313.

Campbell EJ, White RR, Senior RM, Rodriguez RJ, Kuhn C (1979). Receptor-mediated binding and internalization of leukocyte elastase by alveolar macrophages in vitro. J Clin Invest 64:824.

Cohen AB (1979). The effects in vivo and in vitro of oxidative damage to purified α_1-antitrypsin and to the enzyme-inhibiting activity of plasma. Amer Rev Resp Dis 119:953.

Cohen AB, Geczy D, James HL (1978). Interaction of human α_1-antitrypsin with porcine trypsin. Biochemistry 17:392.

Crystal R (1980). Conference meeting in Sassari. Clinical Respiratory Physiology, in print.

De Cremoux H, Hornebeck W, Jaurand MC, Bignon J, Robert L (1978). Partial characterization of an elastase-like enzyme secreted by human and monkey alveolar macrophages. J Pathol 125:171.

Dingle JT (1978). Articular damage in arthritis and its control. Ann Intern Med 88:821.

Eriksson S (1978). Proteases and protease inhibitors in chronic obstructive lung disease. Acta Med Scand 203:449.

Feinstein G, Mahmud CJ, Janoff A (1976). The inhibition of human leukocyte elastase and chymotrypsin-like protease by elastatinal and chymostatin. Biochim Biophys Acta 429:925.

Geokas MC, Brodrick JW, Johnson JH, Largman C (1977). Pancreatic elastase in human serum. Determination by radioimmuno assay. J Biol Chem 252:61.

Godeau G, Hornebeck W, Brechemier D, Robert L. Isolation of an elastase-like enzyme from human vulva fibroblasts. Its implication in local elastic tissue destruction. in prep.

Harpel PL (1976) Human α_2-macroglobulin. Meth Enzymol 45:639.

Hornebeck W, Adnet JJ, Robert L (1978). Age dependent variation of elastin and elastase in aorta and human breast cancer. Exp Gerontol 13:293.

Hornebeck W (1980). On the degradation of elastic fibers by elastases. In Robert AM, Robert L (eds): "Biochimie des Tissus Conjonctifs Normaux et Pathologiques," Paris: CNRS 2:115.

Hornebeck W, Starkey PM, Gordon JL, Legrand Y, Pignaud G, Robert L, Caen JP, Ehrlich HP, Barrett AJ (1980). The elastase-like enzyme of platelets. Thromb Haemo 42:1681.

Hornebeck W, Schnebli HP. Leukocyte elastase adsorbed to elastin is incompletely inhibited by α_1-proteinase inhibitor.Submitted for publication to Biochem Biophys Res Comm

Johnson D, Travis J (1977). Inactivation of human α_1-proteinase inhibitor by thiol proteinases. Biochem J 163:639.

Johnson D, Travis J (1979). The oxidative inactivation of human α_1-proteinase inhibitor. J Biol Chem 254:4022.

Knight CJ (1977). Principles of the design and use of synthetic substrates and inhibitors for tissue proteinases. In

Barrett AJ (ed): "Proteinases in mammalian cells and tissues," Amsterdam: Elsevier/North-Holland, p. 583.

Lacombe ML, Hanoune J (1979). Activation of rat liver guanylate cyclase byproteolysis. J Biol Chem 254:3697.

Laurell CB (1972). Variation of the alpha-1 antitrypsin level of plasma. In Mittman C (ed): "Pulmonary emphysema and proteolysis," New York: Academic Press, p. 161.

Lawson WB (1978). The inhibition of proteolytic enzymes. Ann Rep Med Chem 13:261.

Lestienne P, Bieth JG (1978). The inhibition of human leukocyte elastase by basic pancreatic trypsin inhibitor. Arch Biochem Biophys 190:358.

Martin WJ, Taylor JC (1979). Abnormal interaction of α_1-antitrypsin and leukocyte elastolytic activity in patients with chronic obstructive pulmonary disease. Amer Rev Resp Dis 120:411.

Morse JO (1978). Alpha-1 antitrypsin deficiency. New England J Med 299:1099.

Nishino N, Powers JC (1980). Pseudomonas aeruginosa elastase : development of a new substrate, inhibitors and an affinity ligand. J Biol Chem 255:3482.

Ohlsson K, Laurell CB (1976). The disappearance of enzyme-inhibitor complexes from the circulation of man. Clin Sci Molec Med 51:87.

Omura S, Nakagawa A, Ohno H (1979). Structure of elasnin a novel elastase inhibitor. J Amer Chem Soc 101-15:4386.

Powers JC, Gupton BF, Harley AD, Nishino N, Whitley RJ (1977). Specificity of porcine pancreatic elastase, human leukocyte elastase and cathepsin G : inhibition with peptide chloromethylketones. Biochim Biophys Acta 485:156.

Robert L, Bellon G, Hornebeck W. Characterization of different elastases. Their possible role in the genesis of emphysema. Clin Resp Physiol, in print.

Seemüller U, Meier M, Ohlsson K, Müller HP, Fritz H (1977). Isolation and characterization of a low molecular weight inhibitor (of chymotrypsin and human granulocytic elastase and cathepsin G) from Leeches. Z Physiol Chem 358:1105.

Starkey PM, Barrett AJ (1977). α_2-macroglobulin, a physiological regulator of proteinase activity. In Barrett AJ (ed): "Proteinases in mammalian cells and tissues," Amsterdam: Elsevier/North-Holland, p. 663.

Stone PJ, Lucey EC, Calore JD, Powers JC, Snider GL, Franzblau C (1979). The moderation of elastase induced emphysema in hamsters by post-treatment with a chloromethylketone elastase inhibitor. Fed Proc 119:364.

Umezawa M, Aoyagi T (1977). Activities of proteinase inhibitors of microbial origin. In Barrett AJ (ed): "Proteinases in mammalian cells and tissues," Amsterdam: Elsevier/

North-Holland, p. 637.

Werb Z, Gordon S (1975). Elastase secretion by stimulated macrophages. J Exp Med 142:361.

White R, Janoff A, Dearing R (1978). Inhibition of mouse macrophages, human leukocyte and porcine pancreatic elastase by desmosine. Amer Rev Resp Dis 117:192.

White R, White J, Janoff A (1979). Effects of cigaret smoke on elastase secretion by murine macrophages. J Lab Clin Med 94:490.

Yoshida A, Yu SY (1979). In vivo suppression of elastase emphysema in hamsters by α_1-antitrypsin or elastatinal. Fed Proc 38:1205 (abs. 5161).

Author Index

Subject Index